TRUE STORIES FROM THE ROLLING BAND-AID BOX

A collection of true stories as told by professional firefighter/paramedic John Wyatt after 30 years of responding to 911 calls

Copyright © 2022 by John Wyatt

All rights reserved. No part of this book may be reproduced in any form without written permission.

Printed in the United States of America

ISBN: 979-8-4030-1355-0

Table of Contents

CHAPTER ONE: JUST RELAX	1
CHAPTER TWO: IT'S STUCK	5
CHAPTER THREE: TAR AND FEATHERS	19
CHAPTER FOUR: THE WICKED WITCH	37
CHAPTER FIVE: THE GLAMOROUS LIFE	51
CHAPTER SIX: HAPPY NEW YEAR	59
CHAPTER SEVEN: AX TO THE FACE	69
CHAPTER EIGHT: BOXES	85
CHAPTER NINE: FIREFIGHTER	93
CHAPTER TEN: UNDER FIRE	103
CHAPTER ELEVEN: FINS AND SNOWMOBILES	111
CHAPTER TWELVE: UP, UP, AND AWAY	129
CHAPTER THIRTEEN: 9/11	141
CHAPTER FOURTEEN: IT'S A BAD ONE	145
CHAPTER FIFTEEN: FUN AND GAMES	155
CHAPTER SIXTEEN: WOUNDED COWS	165
CHAPTER SEVENTEEN: THE IMPACT	175

Acknowledgments

I would like to thank Dr. Tiffanie James Parker of Phoenix Blue Academic Editing for all the help she provided this first-time writer. Her guidance and knowledge of the editing and publishing process were invaluable.

I would also like to thank my good friend Richard Hanson. His advice and feedback helped me find my voice in the telling of these stories.

Last but not least, I would like to thank my wife Marie for 30 years of being the wife of a firefighter. While I worked 24, and sometimes 96 or more hours at a time, she worked a full-time job, dealt with home emergencies, and raised two wonderful kids. Our spouses send us off to do a job they know puts us in harm's way, and for that, they deserve our respect.

Dedication

This book is dedicated to my friend and brother, firefighter Shannon Hamilton. He exemplifies the words sewn onto the patch at our shoulder, *duty, honor,* and *service*. Like all the firefighters, emergency medical technicians, and first responders, both professional and volunteers, who serve their communities every day, he has earned and deserves respect.

Foreword

As a firefighter and paramedic, I often gave tours of the fire station to families and groups of children. I would show them the living area, kitchen, and dorm rooms, with another firefighter following at the back of the pack to corral the stragglers. I always saved the best for last, the engine bay. Depending on the size of the station, there could be one fire engine or two fire engines, a ladder truck, several ambulances, a chief's vehicle, hazmat truck, brush rig, a water rescue boat, or any combination of these. Arriving at the ambulance, I would show them the contents of the outside compartments and all the equipment inside. My favorite was blowing up a latex glove like a balloon and drawing a face on it as a gift to the children. My goal was to make the inside of an ambulance a non-threatening place in case they were ever transported in one. I would tell them, "It's just a big rolling Band-Aid box." Thus, the title of my book. In the 30 years that I worked in the Emergency Medical Service, I must have responded to over a thousand calls, most of them just blurring together. The cardiac arrests, strokes, vehicle accidents, stabbings, shootings, overdoses, assaults, house fires, and all the rest are a jumble in my mind. However, the stories in this book have remained clear, as if they have been burned into my hard drive.

It's a truth that firefighters are always on the job, even when they're not. Just because we finish a shift doesn't mean we stop being firefighters. The training we receive gives us the confidence to throw ourselves into nearly any emergency when the men and women in uniform have yet to arrive. For example, I was driving my family up the mountain for a day on the slopes, volunteering with ski patrol, and looking forward to making tracks in the snow with my kids. Coming down the road, in the opposite direction, was a van that suddenly began to swerve back and forth across the highway like a speeding snake. The swerves increased in size until two tires on one side caught on the pavement and the vehicle launched into the air sideways, flipping one complete rotation without touching the road. It landed back to earth on all four tires, rolled into a bank of dirt at the shoulder, and came to a stop.

"Oh my God," my wife says. "We have to stop."

She knows me well. I pull off the road and start walking up the hill, watching as traffic above the accident stops in the middle of the highway. The doors on one of the cars fly open, and two young men come racing down the road to the van, reaching the open driver's window just ahead of me.

"It's okay," one of them says with a bit of bravado. "We're EMTs."

"Cool," I responded. "I'm a paramedic."

You would think I had just told them I was Superman the way they backed away. Looking into the window, I see a woman that appears to be in her 50's sitting calmly at the steering wheel, looking out her windshield. The first thing I notice is that her shoulder-length wig has slid around and is sitting sideways on her head, hair covering one eye. In a quiet voice, I say, "Excuse me, ma'am, are you alright?" Her head turns at my voice. "Of course, why shouldn't I be?"

"Well, you just flipped your van."

She seems to process that sentence for a moment then says, "No, I didn't."

"Ahh, yeah, you did."

Turns out, she was just having a diabetic moment that was easily fixed when the ambulance arrived. The point is that there were three first responders that witnessed the accident, and we all came forward to help a stranger.

As of the writing of this book, it's estimated that there are approximately 1,216,400 firefighters in the U.S. Of those active firefighter personnel, 34 percent are career firefighters, 54 percent are volunteers, and 12 percent are classified as paid per call. Each one of those men and women has their own stories, their own battles. These are mine.

CHAPTER ONE

JUST RELAX

I joined the military fresh out of high school and became a United States Army paratrooper, jumping out of planes and creeping through the steaming jungles of Panama. The training prepared me to enter civilian life ready to hunt people like prey, clean an M16 in the dark, and fall asleep anywhere, any place, and at any time. These skills, to my disappointment, were not to be found on many job applications. *What was I going to do for the rest of my life?* I drifted around landing work like an armored car guard and a bellman at a fancy hotel, none of which offered a challenge that could keep my attention. Then, one night, while nursing a warm beer at a house party, a good friend mentioned that she was in an EMT (emergency medical technician) class.

True Stories from the Rolling Band-aid Box

"What's an EMT?" I asked. We stood together in the dark, crowded apartment while she told me how she was going to work on an ambulance, running red lights, and saving people. Now that sounded like something I could get into, and I became excited by the idea of becoming an EMT. *Money For Nothing* was blaring from the speakers, but I barely heard it because the path of my life was about to change forever. The following day, I contacted her instructor. They were a week into the class but, after a little begging, he gave me a pass, and just like that, I was learning how to treat diabetics and deliver babies. The course was divided into classroom time and practical experience working in a small hospital emergency room. It was an eye-opener.

I'm assigned to a small hospital emergency room in San Diego. On this sun-drenched day, my regular routine of making beds and emptying bedpans is interrupted by a huge African

John Wyatt

American gentleman who comes in complaining of a painful hemorrhoid. When I say huge, this guy could be the Hulk's stuntman. His muscles have muscles. The doctor asks me to assist with the patient in exam room two. The Hulk is lying face down, and the goofy hospital gown can't contain his bulk, exposing his rear. His discomfort is obvious, whether from the swollen hemorrhoid, the fact that he is so exposed, or both, I can't say. My job, the doctor informs me, is to hold the butt cheeks apart so he can get to the offending growth. As diplomatically as I can, I tell the patient what I will be doing. A grunt is the answer I received in response. No sooner than I place my gloved hands on his two well-muscled butt cheeks, he clenches them like an iron vise.

Using the most understanding voice I can muster, I whisper in his ear, "You need to relax." We both take a deep breath, and I spread them wide, exposing a large, very angry-looking hemorrhoid. The doctor injects the lidocaine, which we all know hurts like the dickens, and the patient nearly levitates off the hospital bed. Determined to do the job I've been given, I get a better grip, set my feet in a wider stance, and spread them again. With his scalpel, the doctor makes one smooth cut, releasing a gush of blood and puss. The results are immediate, and the gentleman lets out a long sigh of relief. He is much happier, and I'm wondering if I picked the right career. Wrestling with butts was not in the brochure.

My friend finished the course but then decided it wasn't for her. I'll always remember that she started me in this life. After graduating and passing the state test, I began applying for jobs. In the blink of an eye, I was working as a Basic EMT in a large California city on the border of Mexico. The year was 1985.

CHAPTER TWO

IT'S STUCK

The morning starts out like most, washing the ambulance and checking medical supplies. The rig is scrubbed inside and out each morning with special attention to the nooks and crannies where blood and other bodily fluids may have been missed by the quick wipe from the off-going crew. Gert is my partner today. Her real name is Gertrude, but everyone calls her Gert. She's had three years of working on the ambulance and living on fast food. Gert's a good EMT, and I'm learning the ropes under her watchful eye. We're spraying soap off the side of the van when the call comes over the radio for a woman delivering a baby in a sleepy beach community near the Mexican border. The morning sun casts long shadows off the cheap apartment buildings and is already heating up the landscape.

True Stories from the Rolling Band-aid Box

Sitting in the passenger seat means I will oversee patient care. My mind is running through every possibility I recently learned about childbirth. It seems like I was in class just yesterday, then thrown into the deep end of the pool and told to sink or swim. Sure, I passed the course, but deep down, I feel I fooled them all into thinking I was ready to take care of actual patients. The truth is, I didn't feel ready for this.

The dispatch radio informs us that the baby is being delivered. Gert presses a little harder on the gas pedal while my pulse races right along with the engine. We arrive at a small apartment building surrounded by the brown stubble of last winter's grass. My hands filled with emergency equipment, I follow Gert as she knocks on the green peeling paint that covers the door. My first clue that things are going sideways is the door flying open and a guy screaming, "It's stuck." He turns and runs up the stairs, two steps at a time. Despite the heat, my body shivers a little. It may be what waits for me upstairs or the trickle of sweat running down my back as we follow the man through the house.

Hurrying down the hallway, I come into a room strangely empty. No pictures on the walls, no dresser or nightstands, like they had just moved in and hadn't had a chance to unpack. Against one wall is a king-size bed with the white sheets soaked in sweat, blood, and fluids from the delivery. On it, a woman lies naked, every muscle tense, her legs spread wide, and between them, a newborn child. The tiny, purplish torso has been delivered, but the head is still inside the mother's body. A small twitch of the baby is the first sign I see that the little girl is still clinging to life. We go to work.

Gert places an oxygen mask over mom's face, which gives her, and hopefully, the infant, the needed oxygen. I assess the child, doing my best to ignore the strong smell of blood and urine. The child is lying face down, the body limp, and is several shades of blue and purple mixed with a pasty white. A weak, thready pulse can be felt on

her arm, just under the armpit. Okay, I think, *work the problem*. The baby's head is still in the birth canal, and she can't take her first breath with her face buried inside her mother. I know the solution is to place my hand between the infant's face
and the wall of the vagina to create an opening and allow air to reach the lungs. I hesitate, not believing what I see at first. Surrounding the mother's pelvic area is what I can only describe as alligator skin, rough, scaly, and flaking. Thank God my instructor had beaten into us the importance of wearing gloves on every call.

My brain puts the mother's skin condition in the proper column, then, with one hand wedged around the infant's face and the other holding the barely warm body, I tell mom to push. It has been a long and difficult labor, and she is exhausted from the effort. The fear, pain, and belief that her baby is already dead are painted on her sweat-streaked face. The man who led us up the stairs stands with his back against a wall, watching in helpless silence. She pushes several times, screaming and crying with the pain, her legs quivering with the effort. The weak jerks of the tiny body give me the will not to quit. Like trying to solve a difficult puzzle, my mind continues to look for a solution. *It's about anatomy and angles.* In unison, I turn the body and head a few degrees and say, "Push." She screams and whips her head back, spraying sweat from her hair on the back wall. I gently pull the body to the side, and the head comes free. The mother lets out a heavy sigh and cries great body-shaking sobs — no time for celebrating yet.

The little girl has joined the rat race, but she hasn't taken her first breath. I'm suctioning the child's airway with a bulb syringe when the paramedics join our group, like the cavalry arriving to save the day. While I've been working, Gert has been in contact with them, and they have called for the Life Flight helicopter to land nearby. Quickly sizing up the scene, one of them cuts the cord, and I hand the baby off to the other medic. He takes the child, checking for a pulse and breathing. I stand like a statue as the medic begins CPR[1]. After all the work I've done to deliver that little life, all I can do is wait for a miracle, and it comes.

"I've got a heartbeat," announces the medic. Looking through moist eyes, I see the tiny chest moving up and down. We do another quick suction with the bulb syringe, then with me holding an oxygen tank and the medic holding an O2[2] mask at the child's face, we move downstairs and into the morning light. The bright sun hits her face, and the little girl starts to cry. A few hundred feet away sits the helicopter, rotors still spinning, blowing up loose dirt and grass on the school soccer field. A doctor is waiting for us in the back of the helo and gently takes the baby from the medic. By this time, the child's skin is turning a

---

[1] Cardiopulmonary Resuscitation
[2] O2 is the abbreviation for oxygen

nice shade of pink, her arms moving weakly. Immediately, the doctor starts trying to push an endotracheal tube down the infant's throat to establish an airway. All the while, she gags and chokes on the unwanted plastic tube.

After about fifteen seconds of this, I meekly state, "The child has been breathing really well." What do I know? I'm a lowly basic EMT, and this is a doctor — one of the gods that walk the earth. He seems a little flustered, looks around, and finally says, "Yeah, yeah, let's just go."

I jump out, but before I can get clear, the doctor shouts to me over the beating of the chopper blades, "What time was she born?" I shout back the time and quickly step away from the downward rushing of air and noise. I watch the helicopter rise off the grass and fly away with the life I have just helped to save and realize my short time inside the helicopter has left a huge impression on me. That's where the excitement and the challenge are. I tell myself, *that is what I want to do.*

When I return to the front of the apartment, the second medic and Gert are just exiting the door with the mother lying on the gurney, crying pitifully.

"She's dead, isn't she?" she asks me with so much despair.

"No, she's doing well, breathing and everything," I reply.

Her look of disbelief and joy is something I will carry with me for all my days. That incident has stayed with me all these years. Sometimes I think, *What did that little girl grow up to become? How many lives has she touched?* I'm part of that. I was floating two feet off the ground for weeks after that day.

☙❧

Gert and I finish the morning checkout, give the rig a good cleaning inside and out, then wait for the emergency tones to go off. Some parts of the city have a large elderly population, others have gang activity, and still, other parts are just poorer neighborhoods where people can't afford health care. The part of town you work in determines how much downtime you have. A shift is twenty-four hours long, and between emergency responses, we tell stories of calls we've been on or heard about, run errands, or shop for our lunch and dinner. Our favorite pastime is complaining about management, wages, working conditions, dispatch, and anything else we think makes our lives harder. We love to complain. Even with all this disgruntled talk, the truth is that when we respond to a call, we are EMS professionals. The public receives our best because that's the job. A truth that I have always been proud of.

This afternoon we are dispatched Code 3[3], lights and siren, to an apartment building for a 32-

---

[3] A Code 3 response is for emergencies while a Code 1 response is for non-emergencies.

year-old male with chest pain. Gert and I walk into a well-kept home and are hit in the face with the overpowering smell of BenGay, the muscle ache cream. Standing in the living room is a fit-looking young man who seems fine. My first thought is that the patient must be in another room.

"Afternoon," I say. "Where's the patient?"

"No," he informs us. "I called you. I'm the patient."

He has none of the signs I have learned to equate with cardiac chest pain. I ask him the usual questions about his pain, and his answers are very matter-of-fact.

"It's in my shoulder; I've had it before. The BenGay took it away last time. Yes, the same pain. No, no shortness of breath."

I feel a strong, steady pulse. Everything is telling me that it's nothing more than a strained shoulder muscle. Then, about a minute later, while I continue to assess my patient, he falls dead in front of me.

I blurt out, "Holy shit, Gert, he coded."

"What? He was fine."

"I know. Just get the airway bag."

We start CPR as quickly as we can, Gert on the airway and me on chest compressions. I'm sweating buckets by now, thinking I was about to walk out the door, leaving this guy to die alone on his avocado green carpet. Shortly after we start, the engine company arrives with the medics. Using the ECG[4] machine, they find the patient in ventricular fibrillation[5] and shock him into a normal sinus rhythm. *Yes,* I think. *Saved him!* He's transported by the medics before he regains consciousness. I feel like I've dodged a big bullet and vow never to dismiss a patient's pain as something trivial again. The best way to not get

---

[4] Electrocardiogram

[5] Type of abnormal heart rhythm affecting the lower chambers of the heart, causing them to twitch or quiver uselessly.

burned is to work every call as the worst-case scenario.

That night is dark and moonless. In the middle of my chicken and rice dinner that I have been looking forward to all day, Gert and I are called to a home where neighbors heard a woman screaming. We arrive to find the police standing on the road outside. The streets are covered in a low-hanging fog that swirls in our headlights like phantoms. It feels like we have driven into a scene right out of a horror film. The officers have been inside but would rather not go back in. I don't remember the excuse they made, but I believe it was a combination of the smell of shit that is so strong it's a physical barrier and the ghostly moans that float out of the pitch-black house like a demon's song.

"She's in there," one of the officers says, pointing with his flashlight at the door cloaked in darkness.

We slowly step across the threshold, the beams of our flashlights stab through the darkness like light sabers illuminating large holes in the floor and walls. Newspapers and feces cover the flooring, and we must step lightly, like avoiding landmines. A dead, naked light bulb hangs from the ceiling on a twisted wire. Pitiful cries from a back room, like some lost soul, push us to continue searching. In the darkness, we find an ancient-looking woman lying on the floor in the corner of a back bedroom. Like the house, she's covered in shit. A tangled mass of gray hair falls over her face. Her only garment a silk, pink bathrobe, now torn and covered in filth, can't hide the broken leg that pokes from beneath it at an odd angle.

Marge is her name, and she had stepped into one of the holes in the floor last night, breaking her leg. Pulling the twisted limb free, she crawled as far as the pain would allow. For more than 24 hours, she lay on the floor crying for help until weakness overcame her. Since then, Marge was waiting for death and is surprised when the police arrive instead. We assess her injuries and determine that, besides the fractured femur, she is suffering from dehydration. Gert calls for medics while I retrieve our Hare traction device to splint her leg. The medics are not happy they have to work in the hell house, as it comes to be known. Even in her weakened state, with pain medication administered by medics through her IV[6], she still has the strength to scream like a banshee when we straighten her leg in the splint. She tells us that she lives alone on a meager income from social security and that her house is all she has left. She's transported to the emergency room while we return to base to shower and change our clothes that are now reeking of feces. We learned later that a rumor had spread through the neighborhood, insinuating money was hidden somewhere in her home, and a gang had been tearing holes in her walls and floors looking for it.

---

[6] an intravenous line for administering fluids and drugs

CHAPTER THREE

TAR AND FEATHERS

Our favorite hangout is Denny's, where the waitress looks like Pat Benatar, and the pies come with a scoop of ice cream. Ambulance crews sit around the Formica table and swap terrible stories of patients while we spoon in the sweet goodness at 3:00 AM. The ambulance company I work for won the first responder contract in a nice little coastal city and decided to rent a big house as a base for two ambulances and their crews, with no supervision—big mistake! We went wild in the streets, and legends were born. Between calls, we would play Star Trek. Yeah, I know, dumb and not very professional. We would pick a map grid as the borders, and with one ambulance being the Enterprise and the other Klingons, we would hunt each other. Our spotlights were lasers. What can I say? We were bored.

One fateful day a rival ambulance crew from a different company bursts into our station house and, to the surprise of the crew sitting on the couch, sprays whipped cream everywhere. When we return from our call, the creamed crew recounts the raid, and we immediately begin to plan our revenge. The rest of the day is spent in preparation and waiting for the cover of night. We attack at 0'dark thirty, stealthily moving to the door of the rival station house like thieves. I pick the lock and slowly begin to open the door, barely catching a chair that had been leaned against it as an alarm from hitting the floor. It's obvious they are expecting retaliation. Quiet as ninjas, we creep into the house and find two of them in separate rooms asleep. Not very gently, we drag them into the living room and hogtie them side by side.

John Wyatt

The girl in a t-shirt and panties yells at her partner in tighty-whities, "I told you they would come." First, we cover them in sweet, sticky maple syrup. Then we dump the bags of newspapers we had spent the day tearing into small pieces all over their maple bodies. This is our version of tar and feathers. What a sight! Seeing as they are still on duty, we untie them and rush out the door, yelling over our shoulder a warning to never mess with us again upon pain of even more torture.

One shift, someone thought it would be fun to bring their Ouija board[7] to work. The idea was to sit in the back of the ambulance and contact someone who had died on the gurney. I've always had an open mind to the supernatural and believe

---

[7] The **ouija**, also known as a **spirit board** or **talking board**, is a flat board marked with the letters of the alphabet, the numbers 0–9, the words "yes", "no", occasionally "hello" and "goodbye", along with various symbols and graphics. It uses a planchette (small heart-shaped piece of wood or plastic) as a movable indicator to spell out messages during a séance. Participants place their fingers on the planchette, and it is moved about the board to spell out words.

just because we can't see something doesn't mean it isn't there. For example, you can't see air, but it constantly swirls all around us. Well, unless you're in a large city like Los Angeles, where you can see the air, but you get the idea.

It was a dark and stormy night when four of us sat in the back of the rig to reach the spirit world. Corny, but true. It's one o'clock in the morning, heavy clouds cover the night sky, and rain from a storm splats heavily on the roof of the ambulance — still a nice way to start a ghost story. Remember, like all the stories in this book, this really happened.

The bench seat and gurney are splashed with the bright overhead lights as we sit there with our fingers on the edge of the planchette. We ask if there are any spirits with us. No movement. We ask several more times, and the board is silent as the grave. I'm ready to call it a night when the pointer moves to **YES**. I eye the people sitting next to me, and the accusations begin to fly.

"You're moving it."

"I'm not moving it; you're moving it."

"Well, I'm certainly not moving it."

With nothing settled, we continue.

I ask, "What's your name?"

"**R O S E.**"

"Rose, did you die in this ambulance?"

"**NO.**"

"Where did you die?"

"**A T H O M E.**"

"How did you get here?"

"**F O L L O W E D Y O U.**"

That gives me pause, so I ask, "Followed me?"

"**YES.**"

"How long have you been following me?"

"**S I N C E Y O U W E R E B O R N.**"

I wasn't expecting that. Someone had to be playing games. I thought of a question that no one in the rig could know the answer to.

"Rose, how did I break my collarbone?"

True Stories from the Rolling Band-aid Box

"**B I C Y C L E.**"

The girl next to me asks, "Is that how it happened? On your bike?"

"Yeah. I ran into a car on my bike."

"Oh shit," says a guy on my left.

"Wait a minute," I say. "Let me think."

There must be a logical explanation. I need a harder question.

"Rose, what color is my underwear?"

"**B L U E.**"

I sit there quietly, looking around me at the questioning faces of my co-workers.

"Well," the girl finally asks, "what color are they?"

Slowly, I lift up my shirt, reach down, and drag the top of my underwear up.

"Holy shit," yells the guy across from me, pointing. "Blue. B.L.U.E. Friggin' blue!"

"Wow," says the girl, "that's freaky."

"That's it for me," I say. "Someone else ask questions."

We continued with the others asking questions, but nothing was as personal as my conversation with Rose. The next day I went in search of answers. I learned that something called the ideomotor effect was responsible, a psychological phenomenon wherein a person makes motions unconsciously. I seldom thought of that night again, feeling foolish for believing that I had contacted a spirit. I never told anyone the story, and it became a distant memory until about fifteen years later while I was bringing my ten-year-old daughter home from a sleepover with her friends.

"Did you have a good time, sweetie?" I ask her.

In that tiny voice that melts my heart, she says, "Yes, daddy."

"What did you guys do?"

"We played with the Ouija board. I met a lady named Rose. She watches me."

The hairs on the back of my neck stand up, and I lose the ability to breathe.

"What did you say?"

"Rose," she says innocently. "She watches me."

You can believe what you want, but I became a believer that day.

⭐

One hot day in June, I'm assigned to work a road rally in Mexico. My partner and I are looking forward to it. Easy overtime where the speed limit is more a suggestion than a law. Besides, we have lights and sirens. The quality of cars that are racing range from professional Baja buggies to junkers that look like they were found buried in the weeds. We race around the back roads of Mexico in clouds of hot dust, carrying a cooler filled with soda and a bag of junk food, having the time of our lives.

At one accident, the driver is so badly hurt that we call for a helicopter. What arrives is an old chopper, the kind I've seen on the TV show

MASH. They even strap the guy to the skid, just like the show. The helicopter has a weight limit, and I'm pretty sure this guy is pushing it. We all stand back as the pilot gives power to the rotors. Luckily for them both, the helo is parked on a concrete bridge that stands over a dry riverbed. The helicopter begins to rise then drops back to the bridge. The pilot tries again, and again, they fail to take off. The rotors begin to whine as more power is applied. The bird shudders and begins to rise, but as it starts to drop a third time, the pilot pushes into the riverbed. It disappears below the bridge and continues to drop as the pilot pushes it forward and up. We hold our breath as they race just above the rocks and sand. Very slowly, as if cradled by angels, the chopper begins to rise from the small dust storm it created. We all cheer and pat ourselves on the back. That could have been very ugly. The day finishes without anyone dying, and we return to our side of the border, sunburnt and tired.

After one day off, I'm back at work, transporting patients to their cancer treatments and picking old men up off the floor. Of course, they weren't always old men. Late in the afternoon, Gert and I receive a call to help a woman back into bed. We arrive at a nice home with a manicured lawn that smells of fresh-cut grass, and we ring the bell. A very polite middle-aged woman answers the door and leads us to a back bedroom. What we see stops both of us in our tracks. Sitting on the floor, between the bed and the wall, is a young lady that, by my estimation, could weigh six hundred pounds. She is the largest person, living or dead, I have ever seen.

"Are you okay?" I ask.

She responds in a voice heavy with sarcasm, "Do I look okay?"

Alright, it's going to be like that, I think. I slip into a more professional persona.

"I'm John. What's your name?"

"Sam," she answers.

"What happened, Sam?"

Her mother answers the question for her. "She fell out of bed, and I couldn't get her back in," she says, a little embarrassed.

I kneel near Sam and ask, "Are you hurt?"

"No, I just need help getting back in bed."

We assess the situation. This is not going to be an easy job.

Gert asks, "Should we call an engine company?"

Not a bad idea, I think. *We might need the extra manpower.*

"Let's try it on our own first," I say, getting an idea. Then I ask her mother, "Do you have a couple of bed sheets?"

She does and returns with them a minute later. Even though we are both in pretty good shape, I know we can't lift all of her at once. I explain the plan to Sam; then we place a sheet under her belly like a hammock. With both of us grabbing an end of the sheet, we count to three then lift her belly onto the edge of the bed. Sam is now kneeling beside her bed with her belly on the mattress. The next step is to place the second sheet under her bottom. Gert and I get low, and each places a shoulder on a butt cheek. With another count of three, we push with everything we have. It takes some hard grunting on our part, but with our boots sliding on the shag carpet, she finally rolls onto the bed. Standing over her, panting slightly, we feel a little pride at what we have accomplished.

Sam lays still for a moment, then mutters, "I'm facing the wrong way."
As far as we are concerned, it is mission accomplished.

"We really need to get available for another call," Gert says.

Sam's mother saves us, saying, "I can take it from here. Thank you."

"Alright then. Take care and please call again if you need us," I say.

John Wyatt

Not that I was crazy about the idea of a return visit, but that is the job—helping people who can't help themselves. Gert and I return to the rig still feeling pretty good about a difficult job done well when the tones go off on the radio at my hip. It's a vehicle accident, car vs. motorcycle.

The sun has just set, and it has begun to rain. Our headlights drive away the darkness, exposing the road with a shiny black sheen. Our light bar bounces red and yellow off the buildings like a disco. The new rain makes the road slick, so Gert is more cautious with her driving. We find the accident under tall freeway lamps that reveal the bridge overpass with areas of bright light and deep shadow. A car is up against the guard rail facing the wrong way. Two people stand in the headlights, clutching their bodies in the rain. Lying in the center of the bridge, I can just make out an enduro-type motorcycle and, next to it, a body. Gert parks in the road at an angle to protect the motorcycle rider and turns on the side scene lights that expose the area in a blast of brightness and long shadows. She rushes over to the car to check on the two people shivering in the rain while I grab some equipment and go to the side of the body lying in the road. Standing next to him, I cast a silhouette of darkness over the patient, so I moved to the other side.

I can tell he is young, even with his helmet on. Feeling his neck for a pulse, I find none. I zip open his leather jacket, revealing a red stain of blood. Using my trauma shears (scissors that can cut through a penny), I quickly cut open his shirt to find a ragged gash on his chest. Blood is flowing out of the wound like black oil oozing from the ground. The engine company arrives, and I suddenly have the help I need. After removing his helmet, the firefighter and I begin CPR with me doing chest compressions and him giving oxygen with a bag valve mask. In the background, the captain calls for more resources and directs the operation. My hands, one on top of the other, keep a steady pace of downward strokes. I watch as the rain mixes with his blood, covering my latex gloves. It feels like this goes on forever. The rain is soaking my body, dripping off my hair and nose into the open chest wound as his bright red blood begins to turn a dull pink. Finally, paramedics arrive and take over patient care. The body is placed on a gurney and moved into the ambulance. It speeds away, rain sparkling in the lights. I learned a short time later that his heart had been nicked by a piece of the broken fender from his motorcycle. He never had a chance.

We dry our hair with towels stored in the ambulance and with soggy butts, drive back to our one-bedroom apartment the company rented as a base for our unit. Tucked snuggly in our two twin beds, we hope that will be the end of the night. No such luck! At 0230, our pagers go off, and we struggle out of bed, dress, and drag our tired bodies to the rig. The call is for a gunshot victim downtown. Driving Code 3 in the middle of the night through the streets of the city is different from any other part of the shift. The roads are mostly empty, unlike New York or Las Vegas, which are busy 24/7. The scene is easy to find because, like a gaudy carnival, the street corner is lit by half a dozen police car light bars. Pushing our way past the men and women in blue, we find a man lying in his own blood.

The red stain on his white T-shirt stands out brightly under the beams of the police flashlights. Gert and I place him in full C-spine, the protocol under these circumstances. Full C-spine involves placing a plastic collar around the patient's neck that is supposed to prevent them from looking up, down, or sideways. It can be defeated by an uncooperative patient. They are then placed on a long board and secured to it using straps or tape. In the old days, we used two sandbags placed on either side of the head to prevent movement. Years passed, and the sand was replaced with towels, then foam blocks, and even cardboard. He curses and threatens us with all manner of bodily harm during the entire process—obviously a grateful citizen. I'm sure his mother is proud. Sirens announce the approaching medic unit, and moments later, they are standing there with a gurney. It's a short ride to the trauma hospital, but the medic asks me to ride along for the extra hands. We are joined by a police officer who handcuffs the patient to the gurney for safety. The medic contacts the trauma hospital for orders while I spike a bag of Lactated Ringer's, the fluid that will be infused through the IV that the medic will be establishing. Everything moves very quickly, and before I know it, we are pulling into the emergency bay.

While riding the elevator up to the operating room, I realize that the patient still has his pants on. In class, we had been taught that a trauma victim should always arrive at the hospital naked; otherwise, things get missed. I take out my trauma scissors and start cutting at his pant legs. Like unwrapping the last Christmas present, I find another gunshot wound in his thigh. I look at the medics and smile. They just glare back at me. Seems this lowly EMT-Basic has just exposed a mistake they made by finding an injury they should have known about. Nothing is said. We deliver the patient to the trauma surgeon and his team while I stand in the corner and watch them work for a few minutes. Very cool!

CHAPTER FOUR

THE WICKED WITCH

Working for a private ambulance company means that anyone can hire us for medical transport. We often worked at high school football games, rodeos, even concerts. Today, a family has hired us to transport their son from a jail in Mexico, back across the border, to a psychiatric facility in the states. They had tried to get him across themselves, but he had escaped through a bathroom window in a Tijuana restaurant during dinner. A few days later, they found he had been arrested again and was back behind bars. The local police were willing to let him go, but only if it could be guaranteed he would be transported back across the border. It seems they really wanted this guy out of the country.

True Stories from the Rolling Band-aid Box

With a cooler filled with soda and a foot-long sub, we set off for the wilds of Mexico. The journey through Tijuana is crazy, dodging kids selling Chiclet gum and vendors pushing carts filled with tasty burritos. It's Mr. Toad's wild ride with stray dogs. Finally, we make it to the coast road and begin to relax, watching the blue ocean waves crash against the cliffs and sandy beaches. We are blissfully ignorant of the day that awaits us as the small stucco buildings, peeling paint baking in the hot sun, fly past our window.

The Ensenada jail sits in a dusty field surrounded by dusty buildings. We slowly pull into a fenced area and park, waiting for all that dust to settle before exiting the ambulance. There is no shade, as the sun beats down like it's trying to punish us. Men start to exit the building, some in uniform, others in plain clothes. They make a corridor from the door of the jail to the back of the ambulance. I'm getting a little nervous. There must be twenty or more officers filing out of that small jail for one prisoner. After this parade, the main character is revealed in chains that join his ankles to his wrists. He shuffles out with an officer holding each arm, and the shackles make a jingle sound as they strike against each other. Now, everyone looks nervous.

The patient is a white male, about six feet tall, in tattered pants, a T-shirt, and rubber sandals. I stand there and study him as he's brought to a stop in front of me. Those of you who are Bugs Bunny fans will know what I'm talking about when I say he looks like the witch with a tittering laugh who would zip off on her broom, leaving hairpins dancing in the air where she had been. It's hilarious! This gentleman, however, is not hilarious. He's scary as hell. His gray hair is shoulder length and standing up in all directions like someone has been teasing it for weeks. His left eye is blood red, and a large hook nose sits over a mouth that is missing more than a few teeth, with the ones that are left being sickly brown. He seems unable to stand still, shuffling from one foot to the other and swiveling his head left and right like he's planning an escape.

"Could you place him on the gurney?" I ask.

A few words in Spanish are spoken, and our patient is swarmed. Several men hold him as the chains are quickly removed, then he is lifted into the air by four men, one on each extremity, and placed on the gurney. They hold him there as I secure him with leather restraints — one on each wrist and ankle. Just to be sure, I tie a rolled sheet across his chest and thighs. These will prevent him from lunging up at us. All the while, he brags about how he will escape.

When I'm happy with my work, I say to him, "Okay. Go ahead. Escape."

He bucks and struggles against the restraints for a few moments, then says, "Not bad."

John Wyatt

"We got it from here," I say to the police. With a collective sigh, they break up and, in a cloud of dust, return to the jail. No paperwork, no instructions, we are suddenly on our own. The patient is loaded, and my partner gets in the back for the ride to the border. Tony is new and in training, so I drive.

After only half an hour, Tony sticks his head out of the crawl space between the box or back of the ambulance and the cab.

"I can't handle this anymore, man."

"What are you talking about?" I ask.

"This guy is freaking me out, man."

"What do you mean?"

"First, he's bragging about the kids he's raped; then he's crying about how they beat him in jail. Now he says he's with the CIA, and he knows my name, and he's going to kill me and my family. He's freaking me out, man."

"Okay. I'll talk to him."

I pull the rig onto the dirt at the side of the road, walk to the rear, and enter the box from the double doors. Sitting on the bench seat, I get right in his face.

"Hey," I say in a loud voice, "what the hell is going on back here?"

As meek as a lamb, he says, "Nothing."

"Well, that's not what I hear. Have you been threatening my partner?"

"No," he almost whispers.

"I don't want to hear another word out of you. Understand?"

"Yes."

"Don't make me come back here again."

"Okay."

I head back to the cab. Tony looks at me with his eyes wide, mouth hanging open. The patient is totally silent as we resume our journey. It only takes five minutes, and I can hear him murmuring.

I yell back, "Do I hear talking back there?"

"No, sir," he replies.

Two minutes later, again with the murmuring.

"Hey. Do you want me to come back there?"

"No, sir," he says again.

A few moments later, Tony's head is back in the crawl space. "He's at it again, man. I can't handle this shit."

"Okay. You drive; I'll sit with him. We have a rapport."

Again, I pull to the side of the road, and this time Tony and I switch places.

"Thanks, man," Tony says to me as we pass each other.

I settle in on the bench seat, and the patient starts to talk. The stories are both fantasy and horror. He admits to liking small boys, cries when talking about how the police beat him, making his eye bleed, and continues to brag about being a member of the CIA. I sit quietly and let him talk. It's obvious that his mind is sick, and I'm glad we're headed to a place where he can get needed help. He pleads with me to remove the restraints.

"I don't want to go home tied up like an animal," he cries.

"I'm sorry," I say calmly. "You know I can't do that."

Arriving at the border crossing, I step out of the rig and call dispatch to report our progress and confirm that the hospital is ready for our patient. The boss gets on the phone and says, "The doctor is refusing to take him against his will."

"What?" I say, totally flabbergasted.

"They won't take him against his will. You'll have to let him go."

"No way I'm just going to turn this psycho loose."

"Well, you can't bring him across in restraints."

"Okay, but they will take him if he comes along of his own free will?"

"Yes, that's what the doctor said."

John Wyatt

"Right. I'll get back to you."

Returning to my patient, I developed a plan. "Alright, I'm willing to make a deal with you. If you promise to be good and go to the hospital, I'll take the restraints off."

I look at him hard, holding my breath for the answer.

"Yes, I'll be good. I promise."

"And you'll go to the hospital?"

"Yes, I'll go."

Gotcha.

Tony has been listening and whispers to me, "Are you crazy?"

"It's the only way to get him across," I whisper back.

I call the boss back. "We're on our way. He's going voluntarily."

"Okay," he says, with caution in his voice. "Be careful."

I remove the restraints but not the seatbelts.

"Those have to stay on," I say. "It's the law."

I sit near the back doors to block his escape, holding a large C-cell flashlight in my hands.

I need to stay alert. This guy could get physical in the blink of an eye.

We roll across the border and continue on our way. I try to keep the conversation neutral, but every now and then, he starts to play with his seat belt as if to unbuckle it.

"Hey," I say in my most authoritative voice, "don't touch that."

He immediately lets it go like the boy that gets caught in the cookie jar. This happens a few times, but the situation never gets out of control. At long last, we arrive at the clinic, and the patient even walks through the doors without incident.

"That was crazy," Tony says as we drive back to base.

"Yeah, that was different," I agree.

John Wyatt

I'm spent after so many hours of stress—tired and happy that we delivered our patient where he needed to be without anyone getting hurt. To this day, that was one of the craziest calls I ever worked.

The human body is an amazing mechanism that is very mechanical and resilient in some respects, able to sustain massive trauma and survive. Remember in the Terminator film when Arnold's arm is damaged, and he pulls on an exposed metal rod that activates the fingers of his hand? I saw something very similar to that; only instead of metal, I could see tendons sliding back and forth as the patient moved his fingers. It reinforced just how mechanical we are. The human body can also fail with only small changes in oxygen saturation, blood sugar, temperature, chemical levels, and hundreds of other biological changes. It's the brain that runs this delicate process of life. Weighing in at about three pounds,

True Stories from the Rolling Band-aid Box

it contains around one hundred billion neurons and can do things that seem magical.

Most of us have experienced a paper cut. A small slice on a finger that can produce curse words from the best of us. Afterward, it seems that particular finger is used more than any other, bringing renewed stabs of agony with every touch. What if I told you that the brain could turn off pain or at least ignore it?

Our unit is called to a man that has fallen off a ladder in the mall. We find a construction worker lying at the base of a ladder that appears conscious, alert, and in no distress. I approach and kneel next to him.

"How are you doing?"

"I'm okay. Fell on my back. It knocked the wind out of me, but I'm fine now."

"Tell me about the fall. Did you get dizzy or anything?"

"No, I just lost my footing."

I look at the ladder that is about ten feet tall.

"How high were you when you fell?"

"About at the top."

"Do you have any pain?"

"No. I did hear a squishy sound when I hit the floor."

Confused, I ask, "Squishy sound?"

"Yeah. It was really weird."

My partner has been holding the patient's head this whole time. Intrigued, I inspect the patient from the head down, looking for abnormalities, and I find one. His Pendleton shirt is disappearing into a hole in his back. It's a fairly large hole and deep enough that most of my finger is able to fit when I explore the depth of it. I open the front of his shirt and see the end of a Phillips screwdriver exiting the flesh of his abdomen.

"Ah, listen, buddy," I say slowly. "You've got a screwdriver in your body."

"What?" He says, confused, looking down to see the Philips head sticking out of his belly.

"Wow, look at that!"

"You didn't know it was there?" I ask, amazed.

"No idea."

When he fell off the ladder and hit the ground, the screwdriver had entered his body with the handle of the tool dragging his shirt into the hole in his back. His brain had said, *Nope, not going to feel that, just going to shut that pain off.* I'm sure if he had hit his thumb with a hammer, he would have cursed in pain, but a screwdriver through his body, nothing. He was transported by medics as a trauma and did very well. The tool and shirt tamponade the wound and kept bleeding to a minimum.

CHAPTER FIVE

THE GLAMOROUS LIFE

After two years as an EMT Basic, I felt ready for a new challenge. I had been thinking about Paramedic school for a few months and decided it was time. In 1987, I enrolled in the UCSD[8] Paramedic program. It was the second toughest training I had ever taken, right behind paratrooper jump school. Every day, we would take a test on what we had learned the day before. If you received less than an 80% on any three tests, you failed the course. We lost a lot of people. I would study in the morning, go to class, take a test, then learn new material. After class, I would eat, nap, and go to my job as a

---

[8] University of California, San Diego

security guard watching over an industrial building at night. It was a good place to spread out my study cards on the day's lessons. Every hour, I would do my rounds then return to my studies. After work, I would head home, nap for a couple of hours, then start all over again. This was my life for seven months.

I began my paramedic career with Hartson ambulance in San Diego. The company that made our custom-fitted jump suits also made the flight suits for the top gun pilots out of Miramar air station. I felt pretty cool in my shiny new paramedic outfit, ready to give orders to basics and save lives, only I wasn't. Like a repeat after EMT-Basic training, I had fooled everyone into believing I was ready for this when in truth, I was scared shitless. Thank all the EMS[9] gods; I was placed with a veteran paramedic to ensure I didn't

---

[9] Emergency Medical Services

push the wrong drug or splint the wrong leg during those first few months. If you are old enough to remember Johnny and Roy on the TV show Emergency, it was a 'Mother may I' system. We couldn't even start an IV without getting orders from a nurse over the same bright orange radio. Things got exciting. We responded to more emergencies and fewer 'I've fallen and can't get up' calls.

My partner's name is Frank, and we're having breakfast at his favorite mom-and-pop restaurant where he doesn't need a menu, and they don't need to ask what he's having because he always has the same meal. I, however, need a menu, and I'm just about to order when the radios on our hips blurt out dispatch tones.

"Medic four, respond to a man down in the alley at Fourth and Shasta."

Frank tells the waitress we'll be back, and I follow him to the ambulance. We arrive to find a gentleman lying next to a dumpster, a grocery cart nearby holding all his earthly possessions. We almost miss him, he blends in so well with the garbage, but the smell gives away his position. He's dressed in tattered clothing and worn-out shoes, his gray hair falling in ratted strands about his face and shoulders. He seems barely conscious as I kneel to check him out. Between taking gasps of air and holding my breath, the rancid smell of rotting flesh worms its way into my nose. The crotch of his pants is stiff with old, dried urine. Frank decides we should get him into the back of the ambulance to do a complete exam.

Once inside, we strip him of his clothes and expose the horror show. He has been lying in his own urine so long that it has started eating into the meat of his butt cheeks. There are large open sores filled with maggots, eating away at the dead flesh. The sight of it is burned into my brain cells. We clean him up as best we can, start an IV, and transport him to the nearest hospital. Afterward, we put ourselves out of service to air out and disinfect the ambulance. We can't expose our next patient to the smell that is stuck in our nostrils. So, this is the glamorous life of a paramedic.

We never got back to our breakfast that morning. We haven't even finished the paperwork on our last patient when a call comes in for a childbirth in a bar. A woman had gone into labor in Tijuana, Mexico. She hopped onto the Tijuana Trolly that ran from the Mexican border to San Diego and stepped off in Chula Vista. In pain and fighting the impulse to push, she is able to walk about a block then ducks into the first open door she finds.

It's 10:00 in the morning when we walk into the bar, and I take in the scene. A Budweiser-stained glass light fixture hangs over a Hispanic woman lying on a pool table. The glaring light descending from the lamp highlights her colorful skirt, white blouse, and young face, contorted with pain and framed by long shining black hair. Three or four people stand around the table like ghostly specters in the darkness. I reach her side, tell her I'm a paramedic and ask if I can help her. She shakes her head rapidly up and down, and through clenched teeth, says, "Si." Frank shoos away the bar flies, and I lift her skirt for a quick exam. The bulge in her panties is the child's head.

"She's crowning, Frank," I say, matter-of-factly.

"No time to move," he replies. "Got the OB kit?"

"Yeah, I thought we might need it."

I ask her to lift her bottom and start laying the small blue paper sheets down to create a more sterile area.

It's a shame, I think. *The bar is going to have to replace the felt on this table.* I had seen deliveries before, and they always come with a mess. Things happen very fast after that. Just as I'm getting her panties off, she pushes, and the baby's head pops out, spilling fluid and blood onto the green felt.

Behind me, I hear a man bellow, "What the hell! Get her off the table."

Frank gets in his face. "What did you think was going to happen?"

"Who's going to pay for that?" is his angry response.

"Frank," I yell over the conversation. "still working here."

Frank puts an angry finger in the bartender's face.

"Back off, or I'll have you arrested for interfering with an ambulance crew."

She's pushing again, and I catch the little boy as he slides out. Frank is ready with a bulb syringe and begins suctioning while I rub his pink skin with a towel. In no time, he's crying like a champ. Frank goes out for the gurney, and I give the child to his mother for warmth and bonding. We load the two of them up, and as we leave, I look at the bartender. He is standing at the end of the pool table, hands on his hips and glaring at the mess we left.

"Sorry," I say.

True Stories from the Rolling Band-aid Box

His head swings in my direction.

"Kiss my ass," is his response, and he says it like he means it.

Oh well, I think. *You can't please everyone.*

The rest of the shift is unremarkable—an elderly gentleman with chest pain and then later, a woman who seems to be having a stroke. We treat them, transport them, then wait for the next call. For us, it is just a day at work, but for the people who call 911, it is possibly a life-changing event that would affect them and the people they love for the rest of their lives.

CHAPTER SIX

HAPPY NEW YEAR

It is New Year's 1989. The last day of the year on the medic unit was uneventful. I've been a paramedic for nearly two years now and finally feel comfortable running calls. The unspoken rule is, you're not a real medic until you have worked the streets for a year. My partner, Brody, is new and in training. We have actually been able to finish dinner from start to finish, a feat not often accomplished, and are settling down to watch *Who Framed Roger Rabbit* when our pagers go off. The Border Patrol has requested an ambulance, so we're headed south. Our patient is several blocks from the border fence, sitting on a curb in front of a Safeway store. She is joined on the curb by several other Mexican citizens that seem to be under arrest. The officer in charge gives us the story.

True Stories from the Rolling Band-aid Box

"We caught this group and found one of them injured," he says.

"Which one?" I ask.

He points his flashlight at a young woman sitting calmly. I approach her and notice she has blood all over her blouse.

I kneel down next to her and say, "What happened? Que paso?"

My Spanish is extremely limited, so when she starts to answer in a flurry of words, I can only stare in dumb silence. I stand up and look at the officer next to me.

"What did she say?" I ask.

He gives me a look and says, "She cut her finger off going over the fence."

"What?" I say, looking back at my patient. Kneeling again in front of her, I see her arms are crossed over her chest. I slowly pull them apart. There, wrapped in a dirty, bloody bandana, is the stump of an index finger. The cut is fairly clean, and the bleeding has slowed to a trickle. I'm amazed. This woman tore off a finger going over a fence, then ran several blocks before being arrested. I'm not sure I would be that tough. "Do we have the finger?" I ask. The officer gets on his radio and, after a few moments, says, "Yeah, we got it. I'll take you to it."

We load the woman into the rig, and I follow the Border Patrol Bronco down some dark alleys while Brody treats the patient in the back. I shake my head in mild despair at all the dust the patrol vehicle is kicking up, knowing we will have to wash it off later. These little things make a shift harder than it needs to be. A few minutes later, we reach the border fence. It's about ten feet high, made of solid metal, with interlocking hooks running along the top. It's obvious how she could tear off a finger.

In the pitch dark, at the base of the fence, are half a dozen officers standing in a circle, their flashlights pointing at something in the dirt. It seems that no one is going to pick it up as if it were a live rattlesnake. I grab a zip-lock bag from the rig, walk over to the scary object, and place it in the baggie. The show is over, and the officers split up. The ride to the hospital is quiet. Normally, I would expect crying, but this woman is hard core—not a whimper. It turns out she's a schoolteacher looking for a better life, and I hope she finds it. Not sure if they were able to reattach the finger, but Border Patrol never showed up at the hospital for their prisoner. Maybe losing a finger means a free pass, or maybe the Border patrol is so overworked and understaffed that one schoolteacher isn't worth the trip. I'm guessing it's the latter.

Back at base, we wash the dust off the rig because it's filthy, but mostly because we take pride in keeping our equipment clean and professional. Normally, we would try to get some shut-eye, but it's New Year's, so we drive downtown to watch the drunks. We park at a mall in the middle of the city where there just happens to be a swanky party going on. I roll down the window and open the door to kick my feet up through the open window. We watch couples walking in and out, men dressed in tuxedos and women in sparkly dresses, commenting on how so many of the men seem to be with women half their age. At midnight, we hear the party goer's countdown to the end of the year and cheer, "Happy New Year!"

"Happy New Year, Brody."

"Happy New Year, John."

Another holiday missed with my family, and there would be many more. People begin pouring out of the mall; more than a few are staggering.

At 12:04 AM, our radio goes off for a pedestrian struck by a vehicle. The location is near the border, and I'm surprised that there isn't another medic unit between us and the accident. Brody drives with greater caution, aware that there are more than the normal number of drunk drivers on the road. The scene on the I-5 freeway is lit up like a Christmas tree by lights from Police, Fire, and EMS rigs. We slow down and drive around the vehicles that have closed off half the lanes. Now I realize why we were called from so far away. There are already three other medic units on the scene because there are multiple victims.

Let me explain how a multi-patient scene works, at least, how it worked in 1989. The first medic unit technician is usually in charge of patient care. They locate every victim and triage them into four categories: morgue, immediate, delayed, and minor. As other EMS units arrive, they are given patients to treat and transport. There's a lot more to it, but that's another book by itself. It just so happens that Frank is the lead on this accident. I haven't seen him in nearly a year, but now isn't the time to catch up. He points me to a patient and gives me a quick rundown of the injuries.

"He's male, about twenty years old, head laceration with an avulsed right eye, bruising on his chest, possible hip fracture, and right leg open fracture. You're going to Mercy hospital."

"Got it, Frank," I say and head over to the victim with Brody and our gurney.

Two EMT basics and a firefighter are already working on getting our patient ready for transport. A cervical collar had been placed around his neck, and he is being secured to a backboard. A large trauma bandage is wrapped around his face, and I can see the end of a bone sticking out of a pant leg.

"Good job, guys," I say to the group. "Let's get him loaded. I'll do everything en route."

We work quickly. Everyone is well-trained and understands what needs to be done. I ask the firefighter to drive the rig so that Brody and I can work in the back. After telling his captain what's going on, he's in the driver's seat, and we're on our way, pushing vehicles to the side of the road with our lights and siren. In the back, I'm on the radio to the hospital, and Brody is using his trauma shears to remove all the patient's clothing. I get orders for two large-bore IVs and start to work. Even with two paramedics working on one patient, there is much to be done all at once — blood pressure, O2 saturation[10], oxygen mask, spike two IV bags and start two IVs, ECG monitor, wound treatment, and continue checking vital signs during the entire transport.

    I slowly remove the trauma bandage over his face. I'm happy to find they placed some moistened gauze over the area before applying the dressing. The moistness helps to prevent the gauze from sticking to the blood and other fluids. His right orbital area has been fractured, and his eyeball has fallen out of its socket. Luckily, the

---

[10] The specific balance of oxygen in the blood

eyeball is still intact, hanging on his cheek by nerves and other vessels. I gently place some new, moist, sterile gauze over the area and cover it with a bulky dressing. Brody has cut away the rest of the pants and exposed the open fracture. It looks pretty clean, just a tibia bone sticking out of the leg with very little blood. He covers that with some moist sterile gauze and a trauma dressing. I'm worried about the chest bruise and keep checking his lung sounds, watching the rise and fall of his chest, and checking the ECG monitor for heart arrhythmias. I can't feel any broken ribs, and the patient can't tell me about his pain because he's unconscious.

Since Brody is in training, I ask him, "Is there anything else we can do?"
He answers, "IV, O2, monitor. I guess, just keep updating his vital signs and watch for anything getting worse."

"How about we put a blanket on him to keep him warm?" I say.

"Good idea," Brody says, grabbing one out of the cabinet and spreading it on the patient.

Minutes later, we arrive at the hospital and take the patient straight up to trauma surgery. This time, I'm the one giving a report to the trauma surgeon while everyone stands and listens. Later, I learned that our patient had been one of five Mexican citizens crossing the border illegally. While running across the road, they had been struck by a vehicle at freeway speeds. Three had been critical, one was minor with a broken arm, and one had died instantly on the pavement. The woman driving had been lucky. Her airbag had deployed, and she came away with a broken wrist—hell of a way to start the new year.

CHAPTER SEVEN

AX TO THE FACE

People often wonder why a fire truck arrives at their house when they call for an ambulance. There are usually more fire trucks in an area than medic units, and since a majority of 911 calls are for medical emergencies rather than fires, all firefighters are trained in first aid. Some are even paramedics. These firefighters can begin patient care long before a medic unit arrives. Another reason is the extra hands. Calls like a cardiac arrest or vehicle accident require a large group of trained people to mitigate. There is also safety in numbers.

A fire company was called to a 'check patient' on a freeway overpass. A man had been seen lying on the sidewalk and seemed to be unconscious. The firefighters arrive, and the airhorn treatment is used to determine his level of consciousness. Oftentimes, homeless people will fall asleep wherever they are to recover from their last party, and a blast from the air horn will wake them up. However, this time, it wasn't alcohol but heroin that was responsible for the patient's unresponsiveness. They called for a medic unit and prepared to administer Narcan, a drug that replaces the heroin at a cellular level, thus killing the patient's high. However, the heroin remains in the bloodstream and lasts longer than the Narcan. This means that when the Narcan stops working, the patient can return to an unconscious state, possibly even stop breathing, and die. The gentleman was just waking up from his near suicide when we arrived.

"What have we got, guys?" I ask as I walk up to the firefighters.

The captain says, "OD[11]. We just administered Narcan, and he's coming out of it."

---

[11] Usually a drug overdose

John Wyatt

The patient has heard our conversation and says, "OD?" A female firefighter explains, "Yes. You were barely breathing, so we gave you Narcan to save you from the heroin you took."

"I didn't take no heroin, you stupid bitch. Just had a couple of beers."

I've probably heard the "couple of beers" story a few hundred times from heroin addicts. The patient is getting in the female firefighter's face and seems to be unaware that the four large men in uniform are quietly moving in on him.

"Narcan doesn't work on beer, and you were close to dying," she says.

"Look bitch," he says, poking her in the chest with his finger.

He never gets out the rest of that sentence. Another firefighter and I grab him by the shirt, lift him in the air, and slam him against the safety fence at his back. With his feet dangling in the air, I slowly say, "You do not touch the lady. Understand?"

"Yeah, sure. Whatever," he says with wide eyes. We lower his feet back to the bridge. He's definitely awake now.

"We need to take you to the ER until the heroin is out of your system," I say.

"I told you, I didn't take heroin."

"Look, we know you took it. Your arms are covered in track marks."

"Well, I'm not going," he says and starts to walk away.

"Hang on. You're going to have to sign a form."

We do a report on every call, and when a patient decides not to be transported against medical advice, we make them sign the report stating as much. We release the engine company, and I make Brody fill out the report—one of the perks of being the lead medic. The patient signs and takes off, most likely in search of his next high. That's the life of a hard-core addict, one fix after another with periods of conscious hell in between.

John Wyatt

After that lovely start to our day, we ran to a cardiac arrest that was pronounced dead on scene. The family was devastated. TV shows have convinced the public that we save these people all the time. Truth is, even if CPR is started right away, the odds of survival are small to non-existent.

This brings me to an interesting call about a lovely woman I responded to who was complaining of chest pain. She is an ancient pixy of a lady, heavily wrinkled and sweeter than honey. Under a head of silver hair, her eyes twinkle with life and wisdom. She has a little chest pressure, so we do the usual exam and treatments, then begin her transport to the hospital. I'm sitting on the bench seat enjoying our conversation about my children and her grandchildren when she suddenly goes silent. Her eyes have lost that twinkle and are now lifeless, like a doll's eyes. I whip my head to the monitor screen and see that her heart has gone into a ventricular fibrillation or

V-fib, meaning that her heart muscle, instead of a regular beat, is just quivering like a bag of worms. Our protocol states that in a witnessed arrest, we can perform a precordial thump. I make a fist and forcefully slam it down on her chest. Her heart returns to a regular sinus rhythm, and her eyes jump to my face as she clutches her chest.

"Ow, why did you hit me," she says accusingly as she rubs her chest.

"I'm really sorry. I had to because your heart stopped beating."

"Well, don't do that again, sweetie. It really hurts," she says, rubbing her chest.

I feel bad, but I'm also amazed at how well the thump has worked, having never done it before. I reach for a medication that is required after a cardioversion to give her. When I turn back, the doll-eyes have returned. She's back in V-fib. Making a fist, I hit her again, and again she returned to a normal sinus rhythm.

"Ahh, you did it again!" she cries out.

"I know, I'm sorry."

"I told you to stop hitting me."

"I know. I know, but your heart stopped again. I'm really sorry."

"Please, sweetie, don't hit me any-"

Her voice trails off as the monitor shows her going into V-fib again. The glassy look in her eyes has also returned. You guessed it, I slam my fist on her chest a third time, and for the third time, she comes back to the world of the living. It's beginning to feel like elder abuse.

"Ahh, you did again. Why do you keep hitting me?"

This time instead of answering, I push the medication that will calm her heart muscle and hopefully prevent the V-fib from returning. The drug works, and the rest of the transport is just me begging for her forgiveness and trying to explain why I've been beating the crap out of her. She was

True Stories from the Rolling Band-aid Box

truly one of the sweetest senior citizens I had ever treated.

Later that day, we responded to a call that would bother me for years. A woman called 911 with a headache and numbness in her left arm. Arriving at a well-kept home, we find a forty-something female sitting in her living room, two teenage daughters hovering nearby. I kneel down next to the chair and say, "Hi, I'm John. What's going on today?" While I talk to the patient, Brody is taking vital signs.

"I have this really bad headache, and I can't lift my arm."

Her speech seems a little slurred, and she is obviously scared to death.

She says, "I'm a nurse, and I think I'm having a stroke."

"Well then, let's get you to the hospital."

She shakes her head, tears welling up in her eyes, and nods to her daughters, who are beginning to cry. Brody and I head outside to get the gurney.

"We really need to move," I say.

As we return to the living room and load her onto the gurney, I can see that things are getting worse. She is barely able to move. A look of terror is on her face as she feels her body failing. By the time we get her to the back of the ambulance, she's unconscious. One of her daughters rides up front with Brody as he drives us Code 3 to the hospital.

The young girl riding in the front calls back, "Mom, are you okay? Mom? Mom?" Mom will never answer. She died of a massive brain bleed in the emergency room. That call was hard on me. I work with nurses every day, and they are good, caring people. The fact that this patient knew exactly what was happening to her and felt the terror of it in her last moments was a nightmare. Writing this, I still feel the sadness of it deep in my chest.

ॐ

The sun is just beginning to set when we get a call for a motor vehicle accident with three patients. Two other medic units are also dispatched, but we arrive first. The accident is on a long sloping road that ends at the San Diego stadium, where I have watched many Chargers football games. The massive parking lot surrounding the stadium is empty now. As we drive into the scene, I see two vehicles that have crashed head-on into each other. Head-on vehicle accidents are the worst because the occupants absorb all that kinetic energy caused by the two cars slamming into each other. Getting closer, I see a young man sitting on the curb, hunched over, with his head in his hands. A police officer motions us over with a wave of his arm. We approach the cars on foot. A fire engine is arriving right behind us.

The officer says, "It's a drunk driver. He's over there," and points to the kid on the curb. "There are three people in the black Dodge." I look at the car he's pointing to and tell Brody to check on the drunk driver. I can hear screaming coming from the black car and move to it quickly. All the noise is coming from a guy in the back seat.

"Get me outta here," he yells. "My leg is broken."

I take a quick look and, sure enough, his leg is lying at an odd angle. He obviously has a good airway and is strong enough to scream and thrash around in the back seat. I continue to walk around the vehicle. The driver is moaning and clutching her chest.

"I'm a paramedic, ma'am. Where do you hurt?"

"My chest and my neck. I think my wrist is broken too," she answers with pain in her voice.

"Try not to move your head," I tell her. "Look straight ahead and don't look around."

The fire crew is walking up, and I tell them to get C collars on everyone and hold C-spine on the driver right away. Holding C-spine means holding a patient's head in a neutral, forward position. I continue around the car and reach the last patient, the front seat passenger. I stick my head into the open window. The adult female is lying forward, the seat back pinning her to the dashboard. Her head is resting on the dash of the car like she fell asleep there.

"Are you okay?"

The only answer I get back is some ragged, wheezing breaths. There is blood dripping from her face, and I can't see the damage because of her position.

Another medic crew arrives and asks me, "What have we got?"

"We need to get the guy in the back out quick. Get him on a board and pull him out so I can get to this woman."

Everyone is working now. Firefighters are putting the first two patients in full C-spine and on backboards. The third medic unit arrives, and I assign treatment of the driver to them. I get a

John Wyatt

firefighter to hold C-spine on the unconscious woman in the front seat, and we pull the still screaming man from the back. I explain my plan to the crew and slide into the back seat, taking over from the firefighter holding her head. One person releases the seat latch, and we slowly bring her away from the dashboard until the seatback is in my lap, and I see her face, now next to mine. The damage is shocking. I can only describe it as looking like someone had tried to cut her face in half with an ax. The gaping, bloody wound begins just below her nose and continues back, stopping under her ears. Without the support of the rest of her skull, the lower part of her face hangs down about two inches. The wound is bleeding, but not as much as you would expect. She continues to wheeze through the large gash on her face. Handing off the control of her head to a firefighter, I tell the crew to get her packaged as quickly as possible and bring her around to the back of the ambulance. In my mind, securing her airway is the top priority, and I get to my rig to prepare to do just that.

I have put together all my equipment when the patient arrives at the back of the ambulance. Sitting on the floor, my legs resting on the back steps, they push the head of the gurney into my lap. This is a good position for a difficult intubation. I place the laryngoscope[12] in her throat and gently pull up. It's scarily easy because nothing is holding down the lower part of her face. I look for vocal cords in all that bloody mess, but the anatomy looks all wrong. Suddenly, I see bubbles coming up through the blood and have my target. I slide the endotracheal tube down her trachea, inflate the cuff, and listen for air in her lungs as a firefighter squeezes the bag valve mask.

---

[12] A tool used to lift the tongue away from the back of the throat, exposing the vocal cords, and allowing the insertion of the endotracheal or ET tube.

Her chest rises with each squeeze of the bag, and lung sounds are clear and equal. Time to get out of here!

I get a firefighter to drive us Code 3 to the hospital and another to help Brody and me in the back. It takes the three of us to do everything that needs doing. We strip her, looking for other injuries, and start two IVs an ECG, and her vital signs are checked continuously. She must be bagged with oxygen because she's intubated, and we are breathing for her now. She's still unconscious, a small mercy. As soon as I can, I give the radio report to the hospital, and we arrive a short time later. The last I heard, the woman was still in a coma.

Months later, I was called as a witness for the prosecution against the drunk driver. I told them the story I just told you. You should have seen their mouths hanging open.

True Stories from the Rolling Band-aid Box

CHAPTER EIGHT

BOXES

It's not always blood, guts, lights, and sirens. Depending on what part of town I'm working in, it can actually be a little mundane. It is, however, unpredictable, which for me is the best part of working on an ambulance. My soul would slowly die working at a repetitive job without surprises or challenges. Even on the slow shifts, it's rarely boring. I often responded to diabetic calls where the patient was in an altered state of consciousness, awake enough to get violent when I tried to treat them but could not follow commands. Left alone, these patients would slowly go into a diabetic coma, so we start an IV and give them concentrated sugar water for their brain to function normally again. Depending on the size and strength of the patient, this could mean a wrestling match that could bring good money on pay-per-view. Imagine five guys trying to hold down a two hundred and twenty-pound naked man on his bed so they can start an IV, a firefighter or paramedic on each limb, while the naked guy bucks and screams on his bedsheets. I've been part of this scene several times.

At long last, the IV is established, and the sugar is given. Five responders stand around the bed, their uniforms stained with sweat, while the patient's eyes clear, and the fog in his brain begins to lift. Confused, he says those familiar three words, "What's going on?" We explain what just happened, and too often, it's a story the patient has heard before. The spouse makes a peanut butter and jelly sandwich for her husband, with orange juice to wash it down, and we all file out of the home until next time.

If you arrive at work on time, you're late. Everyone understands that they should be at least half an hour early to relieve the medic getting off. The worst is getting a call ten minutes before the end of your shift. Every morning begins with a report from the off-going crew and, when time allows, the ambulance is prepared for the shift ahead. Batteries must be changed; drug logs signed; every piece of equipment inventoried, checked for function, and cleaned if needed. Engine fluids are checked along with brakes and lights. After the entire rig has been examined, it's washed from bumper to bumper. If we still haven't been dispatched to an emergency, we sit at the table and talk about the day ahead—what we want for lunch and dinner, any errands we may need to take care of, or just the latest gossip. When possible, I take a nap, something I never do at home, in preparation for staying up all night running calls. It's very rare to sit and eat a complete hot meal. So much so that it's almost a guarantee that the moment you sit down to a wonderful plate of food, hot off the stove, the alert

True Stories from the Rolling Band-aid Box

tones go off. You shove a few bites in your mouth and head for the rig, chewing as you go.

Many of the calls had me scratching my head, wondering how some people can put their pants on in the morning, let alone survive the day. To put it plainly, people are stupid. They do things to themselves and others that boggle the mind. I'll give you some examples. I responded to a call for anal bleeding. We arrive to find an elderly gentleman lying on the couch. When I ask what's going on, his roommate answers for him.

"He ain't been able to shit for a few days, so I been trying to help him out."

"What exactly have you been doing," I ask.

"I've been using this." He holds up a small stick that looks like it was torn from a tree limb.

"You know, to dig out all the shit."

I look at my partner, deadpan as if to say, "What the hell!" Then back at the guy holding the stick.

"Well, you shouldn't do that."

"No?" he asks quizzically.

John Wyatt

"No," I say, like talking to a child.

The old man, lying on the couch, naked, except for a nasty-looking pair of underwear with bloodstains on the butt, looks on, listening to our conversation. I stand over him, doing my best not to gag at the smell of a body that has not been washed in weeks, possibly more.

"How do you feel, sir?" I ask.

"My butt hurts," is his surly reply.

"I should think it would. Maybe we should take you to the hospital and get that checked out? What do ya say?"

People do all sorts of crazy things the general public never hears about, like that time a mother received a call from her son telling her that his roommate was trying to kill him. She calls 911 but isn't sure of the apartment number. So now, seven people, two medics, three firefighters, and two police officers, are walking around an apartment complex trying to find the particular unit where this murder is taking place. Finally, we hear weak cries coming from a window, and the police break in. There, lying on the couch, is a young man who appears to be semi-conscious. Sitting on the floor at his feet is another young man, sawing at the other boy's ankle with a steak knife. He seems to have sawed through the skin and muscle but is having difficulty getting through the bone. Both men are in their underwear. The police officer rushes over and takes the knife away.

"Heyyy," says knife boy in a slurred voice, smelling of alcohol.

Couch boy cries, "He's tryin' ta kill me." He's also obviously drunk." He cheated on me," says knife boy accusingly, as the officer stands him up and cuffs him. Knife boy is having a hard time standing. The officer is holding him up by the arm, but his knees buckle, and he just dangles in the air.

"Did not," couch boy cries.
We bandage couch boy's ankle and transport him to the hospital while knife boy is taken to jail.

Some of the saddest calls are suicides, a very real problem in this country. I'll tell you just a few I've been to, like the man that blew his brains out with a shotgun in his garage. The brains, lying on the cement next to him, look like red cottage cheese. Then there was the man who hung himself in his barn. His tongue was blue, swollen, and sticking out of his mouth. A troubled father laid in his bathtub (I'm guessing he was trying to avoid a mess for his family) and shot his face off with a shotgun. His attempt failed. By aiming under his chin, he managed to remove his entire face but missed that part of his brain that controls vital functions. He continues breathing, small bubbles escaping from the bloody mess of what used to be a face. Not all victims who attempt suicide die quickly. For example, a beautiful young girl had been dumped by her boyfriend. Her response was to drink a can of Drano, burning through her esophagus and stomach. I never learned if she lived. These calls, and many more, are burned into my memory. I've placed them in boxes to protect myself. Now, as I write them down, I relive the horrors that I had hidden so well. They will have to go back into their boxes.

True Stories from the Rolling Band-aid Box

CHAPTER NINE

FIREFIGHTER

It's been two years since I became a paramedic, and I decided it's time to move up. Hearing that the North County Fire Department in Fallbrook is hiring their first paramedics, I applied. Fire Department jobs are extremely difficult to land. There can be two to five hundred applications for a few positions. In some larger cities, those numbers can increase to over a thousand. The competition is fierce. Knowing this, not only did I apply, I lobbied. I showed up at the fire stations with donuts, not only a police favorite, and talked with firefighters about the department. I even went so far as to run with the chief of the department when he did his morning exercise. It paid off, and I was one of a dozen people hired to be the first ever North County Fire Department Firefighter Paramedics. Before we could start, we needed to learn how to fight fires, and the entire group was sent to a Fire Academy.

Every morning began with a group run, and I would keep the boys in step with some of my old military cadence calls.

Here we go ... all the way ... Here we go ... Everyday ... C1 30 running down the strip ... Airborne daddy gonna take a little trip ... Stand up, hook up, shuffle to the door ... Jump right out and count to four ... If my chute don't open wide ... I'll be a spot on the countryside ... Tell my girl I done my best ... Bury me in the leaning rest.

Ahh, good times! It was a tough academy with a lot to learn and do. Cutting a fire line in a hundred-degree heat was more like working on a chain gang than training. One incident that sticks in my mind was learning to drive a fire truck. It was a simple exercise: slowly pull up to some cones and stop. The atmosphere is relaxed, and we are all taking turns. When it's mine, I'm excited as a kid on Christmas morning. I sit down behind the

John Wyatt

wheel and slowly drive forward. The idea is to learn where the front bumper is and see how close you can come to a line of cones without running them over. There are three of my classmates standing just behind the cones laughing and joking.

I'm about ten feet away and move my foot off the gas pedal when I suddenly have a brain fart. With my foot hovering above another pedal, I ask myself, *Is it the break or the clutch*? I can't remember. Eight feet away. *If I hit the clutch, I'm going to roll over my friends*. Six feet away. With my foot moving back and forth over the pedals, I begin to panic. Four feet away. Now I've even forgotten which pedal is the gas. Two feet away. *Please be the right one*. I pick a pedal and push, not sure if I'm going to roll, accelerate, or stop. With my heart pounding out of my chest, I stop. They never knew how close they came to being run over by an idiot, and I never told them. In fact, I've never told anyone until now.

True Stories from the Rolling Band-aid Box

We graduated and officially joined the fire department. Since we were the first paramedics who had worked for the city, another medic and I were given a blank check and told to buy whatever equipment was needed to make the program work. It was like giving a kid a hundred dollars in a candy store and telling them to go crazy. We spent thousands of dollars and worked with our physician advisor on drug protocols. For the first year, three of us had to audit every single medic report for mistakes, a requirement of the state. The most fun part of probation, and I say this with heavy sarcasm, was learning the name of every street in the city of Fallbrook. I'll never get back the days I spent on that. After working the streets of San Diego, where I would see shootings, stabbings, heart attacks, overdoses, and strokes nearly every shift, the quiet countryside of Fallbrook was … well, quiet.

One perk was the wildfires. Until now, I had never been on one. My favorite was a big fire in the hills that went on for several days. It was large enough that a fire camp was established. Fire camps are cool. They support hundreds of firefighters with amazing meals and equipment. I'm talking steaks, beans, corn on the cob, and hot rolls. This particular camp was set up at a minimum-security women's prison called the Rainbow Camp. Some of the women there were trained wildland firefighters, and they were badass. I've seen them walking up and down brush-covered hills carrying chain saws on their shoulders the way other people stroll through the park. The fire crews would lay their sleeping bags in a large grassy field surrounded by buildings that held the women prisoners.

One night, I woke up in my cozy bag and peered out to see female faces pressed against the windows staring at all the man flesh. It was a little eerie. The next morning, we were cutting a fire break and putting out small fires that had been started by hot floating embers. The main fire was close, and we were working our butts off. The sound of a large prop plane could be heard coming over the hill, and the team leader yelled for everyone to hit the dirt. Without hesitation, we did—our feet, pointing in the direction of the plane like we were taught. It came in low; the thunder of the engines sounded like it was landing on top of us. I was hit in the legs and lower back with a hard slap from the fire retardant it dropped. The red stuff is like oatmeal and hurts when it smacks you.

Another night was spent on the brush rig guarding a home in the hills near the fire line. Our job was to protect the property if it became threatened. The three of us on the engine took shifts staying awake to watch the progress of the fire. I was sleeping on the hose in the back of the engine when the engineer woke me for my turn. The night was chilly and very dark. Miles away from the lights of the city, stars blanketed the sky, and the Milky Way stood out brightly in all its celestial glory. A long line of flames danced on the hills moving up and down, through the canyons and over hilltops. I marveled at this beautiful sight spread out before me, a memory that has stayed with me all these years.

San Diego county was growing fast and becoming like a little Los Angeles, with its traffic jams at all hours of the day and increasing crime. By now, I had two small children, and my wife and I were having conversations about moving to greener pastures. So I began a search for a fire department where I could spend the rest of my career and safely raise my family. I found one in the middle of Oregon. I applied with over a thousand other candidates for seven positions and got the job in 1993. I left for Oregon alone because we still owned a home in California and couldn't move the family. My wife was amazing, taking care of two small children and working a full-time job while I went off to play fireman. Those first months were hard. I lived in a single-wide trailer with another new hire and rode my bicycle to training every day until one afternoon, my wife called and said she had had it. She sold the house and was leaving for Oregon in two weeks. I had to scramble, and I went house hunting. I found a nice little duplex on a quiet street, but two other couples were looking through the windows. I flew to the nearest payphone and called the number on the For Rent sign. I told the guy on the phone that I was a firefighter with a family and needed the house desperately.

"You're a firefighter? So am I," he said with excitement. "The place is yours."

Sweet, I thought.

Over the next two weeks, I worked to get the place ready for my family, whom I had been missing for so long. It was hard going that first year. In California, I had three jobs: North County Fire as a firefighter/paramedic, Hartson Ambulance as a medic, and teaching EMT Basic at a community college. Now I had one job, my wife wasn't working, and we had all the same bills, but we got through it. Even though I had been a firefighter for several years, all the new hires were given fire training to learn how this department did things. After the training, I was assigned a station and began running calls again.

True Stories from the Rolling Band-aid Box

✸ ✸ ✸

CHAPTER TEN

UNDER FIRE

I'm the new guy at the fire station and have a bad case of sleep apnea. This causes me to snore like a buzz saw. The station I'm at has one large room that we all sleep in, so it only takes one night for the rest of my crew to banish me. Each night, after dinner, I pull my mattress off my bed and drag it into the weight room. My snoring doesn't seem to bother the dumbbells and weight bench. I'm working on the ambulance this shift, and we get a call for a pedestrian hit by a car. When we arrive, I see the police but no victim. I walk over to the officer, and he points under a parked car. That's when I see two legs sticking out from under the front bumper. Getting down next to the brown loafers, I look under the vehicle and see a man with his head jammed under the front axle.

True Stories from the Rolling Band-aid Box

"Hey, buddy. I'm a paramedic. Can you hear me?"

"Yeah," he says, "can you get me outta here?"

"You bet. Ahh, how did you get under there?"

"Walking across the street. Got hit by a car."

"Where do you hurt?"

"Well, my head is killing me. My legs and hips hurt too."

"Can you move?"

"Nah. My head is stuck pretty good."

The car that hit him had tossed his body to the pavement, sliding him under the parked car and jamming his head under the front axle. You couldn't make this stuff up.

Turning to the captain, I say, "He's really stuck. We're going to have to lift the car off his head."

"I've already called for the truck," the captain responds.

John Wyatt

For those of you unfamiliar with fire vehicles, a fire engine carries lots of water and hoses to fight house fires, while a fire truck carries lots of ladders and tools to cut, smash, and destroy stuff. There are other common things that they both carry, but that's the short answer. I can only lay on the sidewalk and talk to him until the truck arrives, so I explain to him what's going to happen.

"We're going to lift the car off your head."

"How you going to do that?" he asks with concern.

"With airbags," I tell him.

"Airbags?"

"Yeah, they're really strong and can lift this vehicle easily."

"If you say so."

"When that happens, it's very important that you don't move, okay?"

"Okay."

"You could really damage yourself if you move, so stay still when the car comes off your head. Got it?"

"Yeah, I got it."

For safety reasons, no one can be under the vehicle until after it is lifted, and blocks of wood are placed under it for stabilization. Otherwise, it could roll off the bags and kill whoever is under it. The truck arrives, airbags are placed, woodblocks are ready, and the car is lifted. It only takes a couple of inches. The moment he feels his head free, he begins to shimmy backward from under the car.

"Hey, hey. I said not to move," I say in alarm.

"Sorry, man. I gotta get out of here."

I can only shake my head. "For crying out loud!"

He pushes himself out from under the vehicle, tries to sit up, but goes right back down.

"OW, shit. My hip."

John Wyatt

The gurney and backboard are ready. We place a collar on him and strap him to the board. My assessment in the ambulance finds a broken hip, a nice divot in the side of his head with a possible skull fracture, and an inability to follow simple orders.

☙❧

One of my first fires with the new department was at a thrift store that sold stuff other people had discarded. I was the firefighter on the engine, and together with my captain, we made entry into a large, smoke-filled storefront. In turnouts, wearing an SCBA[13] and dragging a fully charged hose, I crawl through the aisles, unable to see my hand in front of my face. My mask delivers a stream of clean air while I swivel my head back and forth, looking for the glow of a fire. My captain, crawling behind me, urges me on. I keep running into unknown objects because I'm totally blind, but I continue forward until I'm stopped by

---

[13] Self-Contained Breathing Apparatus

what I think is a wall and begin to hear sounds of what I believe to be gunfire.

I think, *Is someone shooting in here?*

On my left, I see a soft glow of red and orange and begin to crawl in that direction. The sporadic pop, pop of gunfire continues. At long last, I can see flames and attack them with my water stream. When the fire is out, we open some doors and blow the smoke out with a fan. During clean up, we find a small gun shop in the back corner that seems to be where the fire started. Looking around, I see bullets that exploded from the heat, sticking in the walls about four feet off the ground, just above where my crawling body would have been. To be killed by an exploding bullet in a junk store would be a silly way to die.

A cool thing about being a firefighter is that every day is different, and you never know what kind of trouble people are going to get into. For example, we received a call that a man had fallen out of a tree and arrived to find him sitting on the ground at the base of the tree. I approach and notice that quite a few bees are buzzing around him. He is semiconscious and looks like a rag doll with his legs stretched out in front of him, arms at his sides, back bent, and his head lying on his chest. His head and back are bloody. I kneel next to him.

"Hey buddy, did you fall out of the tree?"

"Yeah, had to get away from the bees."

I look at the blood on his head and back, asking, "The bees did this to you?"

"Yeah."

"Okay, we're going to get you out of here."

The fire crew goes for the equipment while my partner holds the patient's C-spine, and I assess him. The blood is coming from hundreds of bee stings. He
had been trimming branches on the tree and disturbed the nest. The insects got pissed and attacked. Being strapped to the trunk of the tree, the patient flailed about until he finally unhooked the harness and fell through the branches to the

ground below. I was pouring sterile water on his head and back, trying to remove the blood when the crew arrived with the backboard. We got him packaged and transported to the hospital with an IV, O2, and ECG monitor. I was surprised that with all stings, he never developed wheezing or other signs of a reaction, other than the altered level of consciousness. It gave me chills to imagine the panic, pain, and fear of being trapped in that tree, swarmed by bees.

CHAPTER ELEVEN

FINS AND SNOWMOBILES

Most professional firefighters are on a shift schedule. There are three battalions, each working twenty-four-hour shifts. This means, without overtime or special assignments, we only work ten days a month. Many of us fill this time off with side jobs, and I had a few. Many of them were as a volunteer, and I did them because I loved the work.

For nearly fifteen years, I was a volunteer diver on the Sheriff's Dive Rescue team. This mostly consisted of body recovery, pulling vehicles out of the water, and finding evidence that was thrown into the rivers and lakes. During the summer months, we stayed very busy recovering our drowned citizens. They were all sad stories, and almost all were preventable. I never pulled a body out of a river or lake that was wearing a life vest. They save lives. That's my public service announcement, and here's my personal story.

I'm guiding a family raft trip down the river on a beautiful summer afternoon when our raft drops down into a deep trough. I'm sitting on the back, steering the boat, when the tail violently pops back up, launching me off the raft and into the rapidly flowing water. Even with my life vest on, I'm driven to the bottom of the river and plop onto my butt. Water is pounding onto my shoulders, holding me down on the gravel. I guess I'm about six feet underwater and wonder why I'm not moving. I look around, through the amazing clear river at the colorful rocks. Oddly enough, I feel no fear or panic. It was beautiful. I simply roll over onto my hands and knees and begin to crawl forward, marveling at the colored stones beneath my hands. The moment I'm no longer being held down, my vest lifts me up, and

John Wyatt

my head breaks the surface. My family, who has been desperately searching for me, point and let out screams of "There he is!"

Probably one of my saddest stories happened one Father's Day. I'm working as a firefighter on the engine when we are called to the ponds for a drowning. Two cousins had been with a group of friends, playing in the water, when one of them began having trouble. The other boy swam out to help his cousin, and when he reached him, the panicked boy grabbed his neck and dragged them both down to their death. Our crew, along with others, are ordered to enter the water and search. The pond is about four to eight feet deep, and searching is difficult, but we don't stop. When the sun begins to set, the chief calls Larry (another firefighter who is also on the Sheriff's dive team) and myself over. He asks us to go home and return with our dive gear. After about an hour, we are suited up and ready to dive.

Everyone has been searching in the area that the other boys pointed to as the last spot seen. I speak with Larry, and we decide to move to a different area. Walking out, side by side, until we can no longer touch the bottom, we drop down, the dark water covering our heads. As luck would have it, we landed right on top of them. With each of us holding the limp body of a young boy in our arms, we head for the surface. The brothers, who have lost their sons on Father's Day, are waiting above.

All drownings bring sorrow, and I could fill pages with the stories of men, women, and children I have pulled from rivers and lakes, like the young girl who slipped on rocks and fell into a twenty-foot waterfall. Below is a small pool about forty feet in diameter and fifteen feet at its deepest point. The problem is that she never made it to the pool. Friends searched, and when she wasn't found, the dive team was called. We had been dispatched to this area before for body recovery and knew that the current tended to trap everything in the deep center of the pool. It was here we found the girl's top, stuck in the small branches that swirled in the hole. There is a shallow area at the end of the pool that dumps water into a stream, but it's too shallow for a body to get over. This leaves only one conclusion. The girl is still in the waterfall. During our dive, we found that a large dead tree had floated into the waterfall and became lodged in it. Our best guess is that the girl is stuck in that tree. We check the waterfall the best we can using poles, and we come up empty. The solution is obvious; we must remove the tree from the waterfall.

Using a large tow truck, we stretch its cable from a point above the pool and downstream of the falls. In full dive gear, I place a choke chain on the end of the cable and dive under the waterfall. Wrapping the chain around the trunk of the tree, I begin to shimmy my way up through the falls, pushing the chain as high as I can. It's not an easy job. Imagine climbing a telephone pole with a heavy chain in your arms and wearing dive gear. Now add the pounding of a waterfall on your head and shoulders. When I can no longer fight against the water beating down on me, I pull the chain tight around the trunk of the tree and fall back into the pool. After swimming to safety, the tow truck driver starts to wind up his cable. It slowly begins to emerge from the pool in a long arch. As it gets tighter, the tree slowly reveals itself. The trunk rises from the water, higher and higher until it finally escapes the rocks and falls back into the pool with a heavy splash. With the tree gone, the top of the waterfall drops several feet. Once the tree is secured against the bank, we enter the water and find her body exactly where we had expected it to be. I will save you from the gory details, only to say that she looked like you would expect the body of a young girl that has been stuck in a tree, upside down, under a waterfall for two days to look.

The dive team is called to search for a man who has gone missing on a large mountain lake while canoeing in a storm. The canoe had been washed up on the edge of the lake, but the man was nowhere to be found. Because of the large size of the lake, it's decided that I will hold onto a rope and be slowly pulled in a search pattern. I'm able to remain at a depth of ten feet as I'm dragged through the crystal-clear water. Luckily it doesn't take long to find the unfortunate soul. The bottom of the lake is like a desert with no rocks to interrupt the flat, white sand, allowing the body to stand out like a beacon in the night. I dive down the forty feet and retrieve the cold, pale corpse. People are waiting on the shore, so we place him in a body bag while he floats next to the boat before bringing him in.

True Stories from the Rolling Band-aid Box

People that drown in rivers are harder to find and even more difficult to retrieve. While camping near the river, a gentleman that had ingested more beer than he should have, went to the river's edge to relieve himself. You guessed it, he fell in and drowned. The dive team, along with a ground search team, are called in to find the missing camper. The part of the river that we are searching is crowded with a heavy forest that goes right to the water's edge. It is decided that we will use a raft to float the river and search. It takes several passes, with some people paddling while others wearing dive masks plunge their heads into the water. On the last pass, I find him lying face down in the middle of the river. I quickly pull my head out of the water and look right, then left at the bank to mark the spot. The problem now is how to remove the body from the very powerful and fast-moving water. After a long conversation, we come up with a plan.

John Wyatt

Using two large trees, we stretch a rope across the river and attach a pulley to it. On this pulley, we set up a rope system that will maneuver the raft from shore to shore and position it up or down the river so that we can place it at any point we need. The body is in about four feet of rushing water, and we know that if we pull it up, even a little, the current will catch it and drag it away from us. I'm assigned the responsibility of grabbing the drowned man off the river bottom. I pick the largest guy I can find to join me in the raft, and we begin moving across the water with a crew on each bank pulling the ropes. Using hand signals and keeping an eye on the body in the river, I'm able to position the raft so that the front is just above the corpse. Now with my large friend holding my legs, I place my hips at the very edge of the raft and dive headfirst under the water. I've borrowed a set of handcuffs from a Sheriff. One cuff is attached to a rope; the other is in my hand as I reach for the ankle of the victim. My first dive misses, as does my second and third. The water is so fast that it pushes me up the moment I dive down. I edge out a little more on the raft, and my safety man grips me tighter. With everything I've got, I dive down hard and stretch out my arm. The handcuff snaps shut around the ankle, and I'm forced back up into the sunlight. The strong current instantly pulls the body off the riverbed, and if not for the rope, we would have lost him. Putting our backs into it, we pull on the rope and drag him into the raft. After that, it was only a matter of the crew pulling us back to shore.

For more than ten years, I volunteered in the first aid room at a ski resort. The two biggest perks were my entire family got to ski for free, and no one ever died on the slopes while I was there. I treated many knee and wrist injuries, mostly on snowboarders, and used old carpet foam to pad the cardboard splints. My favorite part was flying around the slopes on a snowmobile to pick up injured skiers. During the off-season, I helped train the staff, teaching all types of first aid.

My friend Larry, who got me into the dive team, told me about Young Life camps. They needed medics to treat the hundreds of young adults that visit the camp every year. Young Life is a Christian organization that brings young people closer to Jesus. These camps are amazing, with water activities, adventures, and sports. Depending on the camp, there may be lakes, pools, go-karts, horseback riding, ropes courses, sing-alongs, and numerous activities run by counselors. The kids live at camp for a week and leave with their souls rejuvenated. I volunteered at the Woodleaf and Wildhorse camps for many years. It was a working vacation for me and a real vacation for my family. My kids were in heaven at these camps, participating in all the activities with the campers. At Wildhorse, the medical staff lived in a beautiful old two-story, Victorian-style home that had been a stagecoach stop in the old days. There was usually a doctor, a nurse, and a medic with their families, and we had wonderful times together. With all these kids running around, there were always injuries. In the summer months, we had campers dropping like wet noodles from the heat.

One week at Woodleaf, the bees took over the camp. There were millions of them, and we often had meals outside. "Would you like some potato salad with your bees?" is something you don't often hear. Another week at Wildhorse, the flu attacked the campers and staff like wildfire. Everyone got sick, even me. I was running from dorm to dorm, dispensing drugs like the Candyman. Not my favorite trip.

One warm summer night, the kids are dancing down at the basketball courts to music blasting from a boombox. A camper goes down with an injury, and I'm called to respond. Driving up in my golf cart, I see a small circle of people, surrounded by a larger group of dancing kids, standing on the court looking down at their fallen friend. Weaving my way through the crowd of dancers, I arrive at the side of a young boy crying in pain and holding his right knee.

I ask, "What's going on, buddy?"

He stares at me with a blank look on his face, then speaks to a friend standing next to us in Chinese. I had heard that there was a group of campers from China. They were supposed to have a translator with them.

"Does anyone speak English?" I say, looking around at the group surrounding me.

All I get are blank stares until a young girl steps forward.

"He hurt knee."

"Thank you. Let's take a look then."

I begin to reach for his knee, and he pulls away. The boy is in very real pain, moaning and rocking back and forth, afraid to let me touch him.

I look at the girl and tell her, "Ask him to be still and let me check his knee, please."

She speaks to him. He looks at me, looks at his knee, looks back at me, and nods his head. I gently feel his knee under his pants, and he winces slightly but holds still. I can feel deformity under my fingers.

"I'm going to have to cut his pants," I say to the girl.

She speaks to him as I pull out my trauma shears and cut his pant leg to expose the knee. The bright court lights expose his dislocated kneecap in all its blazing glory. I speak to my little interpreter, "Tell him I can fix his knee, and he will feel much better, but he has to stay still while I do it." She relays my words. The boy is now staring at me with wide eyes. I can't blame him.

He must be scared to death, I think. *He has no idea what I'm going to do.* I slowly lift his leg and place his ankle under my arm, all the while talking to him in the most soothing voice I can muster.

"It's okay. It's going to be just fine. Try to relax."

I know he doesn't understand the words I'm saying, but I say them anyway. Around me, the crowd seems to be holding its breath. I perform the maneuver that will push his kneecap back into place. He gives a little scream of pain, and it's over. With the kneecap back where it belongs, the boy is grinning like a Cheshire cat. A stream of Chinese is pouring out of him. I'm guessing he's thanking me. I nod, smile back, and get on my radio to request an ambulance transport for a camper to the hospital for X-rays.

Years ago, I saw a scuba diver working in a large fish tank at an aquarium and added that job to my bucket list. After taking the required training, I got my chance to check that one off and began volunteering at the Newport Aquarium as a habitat diver. It was a blast! They have several large tanks with a walk-through tube for visitors. It's one of the best dive spots in Oregon, with crystal clear water and tons of fish. With lots of fish comes lots of fish poop. Therefore, I spent many hours on my knees, in the sand, vacuuming up fish shit. I remember one of my first days, sitting on a ledge above the tank, my feet in

the water, fins resting on a step. I was putting on my gloves when something below me caught my eye. It was a four-foot wolf eel winding around my ankles. Wolf eels have large gnarly heads that look like those dried apple face dolls, only with needle teeth. When you see one, you think that it might likely chew your face off, but this one just wound around my feet like a house cat rubbing my leg. I could almost hear him purring.

    Divers are the biggest creatures in the tank, so we draw a crowd. One of my favorite things was to float upside-down, remove my regulator, then smile and wave at the kids. I often worked in the shark tank, which had bigger poop, a cement floor, and much larger fish. There are several types of sharks, rays, and an assortment of other fish, all with their own territories and movement patterns. The largest is a nine-foot-seven-gill shark with an attitude. One day, while cleaning the top of the acrylic tube, I unknowingly put myself in the seven gill's pattern. Minding my own business, I suddenly feel someone punch me hard in my back. I turn to see that nine-foot bully swim around me and give me the stink eye as if to say, "You're in my way."

True Stories from the Rolling Band-aid Box

CHAPTER TWELVE

UP, UP, AND AWAY

You'll remember the story about the breach baby we saved back when I was a young padawan[14] EMT. I had a brief encounter with Life Flight and many more since then. It was still my dream to work on a helicopter, so when I heard they were hiring, I jumped at it. I believe my experience in the military, throwing myself out of helicopters and working around them, gave me an edge on the competition. I was hired and fitted for a flight suit. Working for Life Flight was a privilege and a great responsibility. We got the sickest patients and the worst traumas. Many of the patients we transported were in remote areas like forests,

---

[14] The word used for a young Jedi Knight

mountain tops, and even ski resorts. It's difficult to describe the beauty of flying through a cloud, soaring high over the city lights of Portland at night, or skimming over the Columbia gorge. A flight team consists of a pilot, a flight nurse, and a flight medic, each with specific jobs. Many of our calls were for the emergency transport of a critical patient from one hospital to another. We also responded to major traumas of every kind that were usually a far distance to the nearest trauma hospital. Occasionally, we would fly to a fire department for a dog and pony show. The crew would teach firefighters how to prepare a landing zone, when to approach the helicopter, and how best to assist the flight crew.

I'm sitting in the co-pilot seat, looking forward to today's dog and pony because it's at the fire department I work for. The sky is a deep blue with amazingly bright white clouds floating past like islands of cotton candy. But,

John Wyatt

unfortunately, my serenity is interrupted by a little hiccup. The helicopter has suddenly lost power, and each time the pilot tries to give the rotors more power, it has the opposite effect.

"We're going down," he announces and immediately gets on the radio. "Mayday. Mayday," he says calmly into the mic and gives our identifier and location. Without looking at me, he says, "Watch for wires and trees."

We're dropping out of the sky quickly now, not like a stone, more like a fat bird with tiny wings. It's enough to put my stomach into my chest. In the back, the nurse mutters something under her breath and struggles to fasten her seat harness. I can't quite make out what she's saying, but I'm hoping it's a little prayer. My head is on a swivel, and I'm thankful we're in cow country and not over a city. The ground is rushing up at us at a rate that makes me believe these may be my last moments of life. Time enough for me to realize I'm going to die but not enough time for my life to flash before me. At the last minute, the pilot flares the rotors up, and the helicopter stalls like it suddenly held its breath. The skids touch down on the green pasture, and we're sliding forward. Traveling about twenty feet, we finally come to rest against a dirt berm.

I'm patting the pilot on the shoulder. "Great job! Great job!"

The three of us get out of the chopper, and the nurse runs around the tail to give the pilot a big hug. It's definitely a "happy to be alive" moment. Now we just have to find out where the heck we are. The nurse and I walk to a nearby farmhouse, open the white picket fence gate, and knock on the door. The farmer is a little surprised to see a helicopter in his field but gives us his address anyway. It takes about an hour for the mechanic to arrive in his little red pickup truck. He and the pilot board the downed aircraft and start her up. They hover five feet off the ground for about twenty minutes, rotors spinning, grass flying until the mechanic finally comes over to tell us to drive back to base. He and the pilot will fly back.

I'm thinking: *You're a braver man than I, Gunga Din.* The helicopter rises off the ground, hovers for a few minutes, and then flies off into the sunset. When the chopper is just a dot in the sky, the nurse and I drive back in the tiny old truck. It's a big change from the sweet ride that got us here, but at least it's not going to fall out of the sky, crash, and burn. As far as I know, they never learned what had caused us to go down, which made me a little nervous. I would much rather be able to point and say, "Oh, it was this little doohickey, and now it's fixed."

The experience did nothing to change my mind about working for Life Flight, and I continued to fly missions for the next two years. Occasionally, a longer transport would be required, and we would fly on a private jet. Very cool and very cramped! I couldn't stand up and had to work bent over the patient. Oh well, the snacks were good.

My last day as a flight medic was both the most exciting and the worst. The first mission was a transport from a small clinic in eastern Oregon to Portland. The pilot flew us over the river through the Columbia gorge, presenting a spectacular view of all the waterfalls. The third mission that day was one I will never forget. We are dispatched to a small rural hospital to meet with an ambulance that is bringing in a ten-year-old boy who has been in a vehicle accident. The boy's grandmother had been driving, and first responders believe she had a heart attack, causing her to cross the center line and smash head-on into a semi-truck. She was pronounced dead on the scene. The boy sustained massive trauma and required transport to the trauma hospital in Portland. We land on the helicopter pad next to the hospital parking area and exit the bird to wait for the ambulance. Standing in the bright sunlight,

I see a doctor, his white coat fluttering behind him as he runs towards us.

He arrives, breathless, and says, "I'm going to stabilize the patient before you take him. We're short-staffed, so I want the nurse and medic to help. Is that okay?"

"Of course," the nurse answers, and we begin walking to the emergency room.

In the distance, we see the ambulance emerge from the trees—lights and sirens screaming their urgency at us. We all arrive at the entrance of the ER together. The rear doors of the ambulance burst open, the EMT jumps out, turns, and pulls out the gurney. The boy looks small, his chest exposed, and another EMT is doing compressions on it.

"He coded just a few minutes ago," says the EMT, as they pull the gurney from the ambulance.

The boy is rushed into the hospital. The doctor directs us to bypass the emergency room and leads us straight into a surgical suite. A dozen things happen all at once. Vital signs are taken,

ECG started, CPR is continued, the flight nurse intubates the boy as I start an IV in the external jugular and look for a second IV site. The doctor quickly decides to open the boy's chest. Under the glaring operating room lights, he takes his scalpel and makes a cut from the top of his sternum to his belly button. As the blade moves down, blood begins to pour out on either side of the body, like a glass that is too full, spilling onto the hospital bed. The doctor begins repairing damaged tissues, the nurses sopping up blood with gauze and suction. Between giving blood through his IV and drugs, the boy's heart begins to beat. We all continue to work. The doctor has sewn all the tears he can find and is now cauterizing all the smaller bleeds. The nurses are still suctioning blood, administering drugs, and doing a dozen other tasks. I've been able to establish a second IV and am looking for a third. He codes again, and we start CPR. This fight for the youngster's life goes on for over an hour. He codes several more times, and each time, we bring him back.

John Wyatt

The doctor finally steps away from the bed and declares, "That's it. I've stopped all the bleeding."

He codes again, and CPR is started. We work on the small broken body a little longer, no one willing to give up, but it's to no avail. We've lost him. The doctor calls it, and I walk through the double doors, out of the room, and place my sweat-soaked back on the wall. My legs are shaking slightly as I slide down and rest my hands on my thighs. My head hangs down, and I say a few words to the dead boy in the other room.

"I'm sorry, buddy. I really am. We tried our best. You rest now. You rest."

I look up and can see the family gathered at the end of the hall. There is hugging and crying. I can't imagine the pain that is waiting for the woman who has lost both her mother and son on the same day.

I worked for Life Flight for nearly two years, flying all over Oregon. It was an honor and the pinnacle of my EMS career. As they say, all good things must end, and my life as a flight medic was no different. The helicopter they stationed in Corvallis had been a failed experiment. It didn't generate enough income and was sent back to the Portland area. Now, I had a two-hour commute and was taking shifts from full-time medics. I asked my supervisor if she could guarantee me a job next month. She couldn't, so I applied for the Emergency Medical Technician Intermediate Instructor position at the local community college and got it. Many years ago, I had taken the Instructor 1 and Instructor 2 courses. Part of the class was to teach a subject while being videotaped. Watching myself speak in front of the class was a big revelation. It went something like this.

"First, you take the ahh, thingy. Then you, ahh, put it in the other ahh, thingy. After that ahh, you ahh, have two ahh, thingies."

Every time my mind paused, I said "ahh" out loud. It was incredibly, ahh, distracting. I still say "ahh" when I pause in my speaking, only now I say it in my mind and, ahh, not out loud.

John Wyatt

For seven years, I taught EMT Basics on how to start IVs, push different drugs, and all the skills required to become an EMT Intermediate. For those seven years, my students had the highest first-time pass rate for the state certification test in Oregon—a fact I'm very proud of. During this time, I also began working for the state of Oregon as a Certifying Officer, running state EMT certifying tests. I know what you're thinking, and no, I was not allowed to certify my own students. However, I must say that I couldn't have been as successful teaching the course if it wasn't for my co-instructor Robin or my supervisor Kathy. I depended on both of them, and they never let me down.

True Stories from the Rolling Band-aid Box

✸✸✸

CHAPTER THIRTEEN

9/11

On the morning of 9/11, I had just arrived at the station house, and the guys were already watching the TV. One tower had been hit, and it was hard to imagine the size of the emergency our brothers were facing. Firefighters don't use elevators on high-rise fires, and we all knew that the stairways had to be filled with people coming down and firemen going up. When the second plane flew into the other tower, it's clear we were being attacked. The unimaginable continued to unfold. The towers fell, people died, and the searching began. About a month later, a few of us decided to travel to New York to honor our fallen brothers. I didn't have dress blues, so a chief officer graciously lent me his.

I had never been to NYC and was like a fish out of water. Riding subways and walking around in circles, I finally found my hotel. The room was like something out of an old movie. About the size of my bedroom at home, it had two bunk beds, no toilet or sink. Luckily, I had a window that looked out at a small, dirty alley. The five of us got together that morning and went to the pile, as it's called. When you first saw the site of the attack, it was difficult for your mind to grasp the size and scope. Massive skyscrapers looked as if a giant hand had ripped down their sides, exposing the floors and offices inside. Many of them were covered with giant sheets of clear plastic or tarps. These buildings surrounded a hole filled with twisted metal and smoke that was still rising from the ruin. You should understand that the destruction we saw was on such a large scale that it didn't look real.

On the edge of the pit was a fire station that had miraculously survived. Walking inside, we met a lone firefighter watching over things. He was young and looked exhausted. The boy must have been working in the pile for weeks, and it showed. He walked around the station, answering questions like a shell-shocked zombie. My heart went out to him. Everything in the station was covered in a thick coat of dust. Firefighter turnouts and helmets still hung in open lockers like gray ghosts, and I realized their owners would never put them on again. Everyone that stood or walked in the station spoke in hushed whispers like they were in a holy place.

The next day, in our dress blues, we began going to funerals. There were two every day, and we went to both. At every funeral, men in uniform from fire departments all over the United States lined up. I even saw patches from Australia. The lines were three to five men deep on both sides of the road and went for blocks. The sound of bagpipes would bounce off the buildings and announce the arrival of the fallen. We would stand and salute the coffin when it arrived, then wait in our lines during the service that was broadcasted over loudspeakers, not leaving until the family had left the church. The station houses were open to us, and they would serve beer to uniformed firefighters. Some of these working stations were like museums. I walked into one where the apparatus door seemed too small for an engine. It had been built to accommodate a horse-drawn fire unit, and there was still a hayloft.

Nevertheless, the city welcomed us with open arms. Attractions like the Empire State building and tour buses were free to firefighters, and many of the bars gave us beer on the house. It made me proud to be a firefighter. To be acknowledged as a brother to those brave men and women who lost their lives saving others. It also humbled me. That level of bravery is hard to live up to.

CHAPTER FOURTEEN

IT'S A BAD ONE

You never really get a good night's sleep at the fire station. Your mind is always listening for the alert tones to go off, and when they do, you have seconds to jump into action. Sleeping through the blaring tones is difficult but not impossible. I've been sitting in the fire truck or ambulance, waiting for another firefighter to arrive, only to run to their room a few minutes later and bang on their door.

"What?" is the usual response.

"We got a call," I would say to the door.

"Shit, okay, okay. I'll be right there."

I won't pretend that I never missed the tones; everyone has. In the larger stations, with several different rigs, the tones may not be for everyone. I've jumped out of bed, dressed, and stumbled to my rig, only to sit there for a few minutes before realizing the tones were not for me. What really sucks is hearing the tones when you're in the shower. Here's a tip, never slide down a brass fire pole with wet hands. Your hands will stick to the pole and burn like hell.

Working the engine one night, we were dispatched to a structure fire. The kind of call that gets everyone's adrenaline flowing. I'm sitting in the back of the speeding engine, getting on my SCBA, when I see the glow of a large fire just off the freeway. *This is going to be good.* We arrive at a large industrial business with flames shooting thirty to forty feet into the night sky. The captain issues orders, and my first job is to set up a deluge gun or fire monitor that will deliver a master stream of water on the fire. I remove the monitor[15] from the engine, a crazy piece of metal tube that bends this way and that like a snake, and start off

---

[15] An controllable high-capacity water jet used for manual firefighting. Also called a deluge gun, fire monitor, master stream, or deck gun.

John Wyatt

across a grassy field in the pitch dark. My only light is the red glow of flames lighting up the sky.

With help from my engineer, we set up the monitor and stretched the five-inch hose nearly one hundred feet to the engine. Later, our crew is ordered to another part of the fire that covers about three blocks of the burning factory. Our assignment is to protect a small metal shed that holds a concrete vat. The vat is about ten feet long, six feet wide, and five feet deep, with twelve-inch-thick walls. It holds acid that is boiling from the heat of the fire. We're warned not to kneel on the floor because some of the acid may have splashed onto it. Three of us stretch the hose inside the shed, putting water on the wall and ceiling. As we duck walk inside, I'm next to the vat. Out of curiosity, I slowly stand up and peer into the concrete bath. Acid is boiling like a pot of water waiting for the lobster. My pucker factor increases to a ten. We extinguish the fire in this area, and I get a new assignment. Three trucks have been parked around the fire, with ladders raised high above it. I climb to the top of one of the ladders to operate the master stream. Below me is the inferno. Twisted metal beams poke through collapsed roofs like the ribs of whales, and everything is on fire. I have a bird's eye view of three blocks of hell spread out before me. I direct the water to different parts of the fire, and steam rises in protest, blocking my view of the carnage below. It's beautiful! We're there all night, digging into small areas, putting out hidden fires. In the morning, we're replaced by oncoming crews that continue the cleanup.

What can I say? Structure fires are fun, hard work, but fun. Most firefighters enjoy cutting holes in roofs, smashing through walls, and putting out fires. One of our jobs during a house fire often requires us to use pike poles (a long pole with a spike and hook on the end) to tear down the ceiling and look for fire extension in the rafters. Being tall, it was fun for me to just punch my fist through the ceiling and pull it down with my hand.

We also like tearing up vehicles. There is something about finding a patient trapped in the twisted metal of a car, then pulling and cutting the crap out of the vehicle to free them. It takes teamwork and training to do it right.

It was just another night on the medic unit when we were dispatched to a vehicle accident. We arrive to find a dark sedan lying on its roof in the middle of the intersection. Police lights throw flashing colors all around. I approach and have to get down on my belly in order to shine my flashlight into the broken window. A man lies trapped in the front seat. The car's roof is partially crushed, with the seat-backs pushing against the ceiling of the car.

I introduce myself and ask, "How are you doing?"

True Stories from the Rolling Band-aid Box

"I think my leg is broken."

I continue asking questions but will have to enter the vehicle to do a proper assessment. I squeeze through the broken window, my turnout coat protecting me from the broken glass that is everywhere. Smells of the wrecked car fill the space. I crawl across the roof to the victim's side; it's a tight fit. The bright beam of my flashlight shows the man's face in brilliant contrast to the darkness all around us and reveals the face of a second victim. Another man lies crushed in the back seat, his body hidden by the front seats. His face, stuck between the headrest and the roof of the car, is deformed. Like a vise that has squashed the two sides of his head together, his eyes bulge. At the same moment my flashlight hits his face, the first man sees the face of his friend, inches from his own, and begins to scream. I quickly turn off my light and try to calm him down, but that vision is too much for him. Even with his friend's face in the darkness, the knowledge that it is so close is a living nightmare. I call for a blanket and cover the dead man's crushed skull. It will take time to remove the injured man from the car. Meanwhile, all I can do is sweat in my heavy coat and talk to him. Eventually, the screaming turns to sobbing. I remain with him until he is freed from the car and then ride with him to the hospital.

As I've said before, you never know what will happen in the ambulance, and this day was no different. We're called to another vehicle accident and arrive to find that the engine crew is already on scene. Before I'm able to step out of the rig, the captain walks up to my window and says, "Get down there quick. It's a bad one." It looks like a normally quiet neighborhood, but today, it's anything but. People have come out of their homes to see the circus.

I'll tell you the story that I received from the police officer at the hospital after the call. I knew very little of the facts until then. A woman was hit by a car driven by a man against who she had a restraining order. He saw her on that bright sunny day, riding her bike, and decided to kill her by smashing his vehicle into her with enough force to launch her onto the hood of his car, then take down a telephone pole, turning the base into splinters. Neighbors heard the crash and came out to find the pole lying on the car along with the woman. Seeing that the woman was still alive, the driver got out of his car, jumped on the hood, and started to stomp on the woman's head. The concerned citizens pulled the man off the woman and dragged her to a nearby grassy field, where I found her.

She's a young woman, not unattractive, wearing shorts and a t-shirt. She lies in the green grass; her long dark hair frames her face. The milky skin of her throat has been torn open, revealing the bloody red meat and muscle below. She's unconscious, and the slow rise and fall of her

John Wyatt

chest tells me she's breathing. As I'm doing my assessment, I notice a man sitting in the grass, ten feet away, legs crossed, staring intently at the woman. I didn't know at the time that this was the person that ran her over. On closer inspection, I can see that she's breathing from the gash in her throat. Small bubbles escape the bloody wound with each exhalation. I suction the area, but the damage is so horrific I can't see where the bubbles are coming from. My partner and I package her up and transport her Code 3. I bring another firefighter along for the extra help. Taping a tube to her C-collar and pointing it at the gash delivers oxygen to the area while I continue to suction, doing my best to keep her airway clear. It's a short drive to the emergency room, and the trauma doctor is waiting at the back of the ambulance when the doors open. I give my report as we quickly wheel the patient to the trauma room. The doctor removes the collar and begins to poke his finger into the bloody mess that had been her throat. Suddenly, the intake of air stops. He's found the hole and replaced his finger with an ET tube. The airway is now secure. They never taught me that move in paramedic school, and I learned something new.

CHAPTER FIFTEEN

FUN AND GAMES

Life for a firefighter isn't all blood and death; we actually save lives, like the guy who hid in his closet while his house burned down. I was on a hose pouring water into a window when a crew dragged his soot-covered body out the front door. He wasn't breathing, and they started CPR right there in his driveway. Moments later, he had a pulse and was coughing up the smoke he had inhaled. All calls are not life-threatening either. I could fill another book with all the silly reasons people call 911.

For instance, one guy got off the Greyhound bus downtown around midnight and called for an ambulance. We arrive with an engine crew to find him standing on the curb with his suitcase. Five guys who had been working all day are now standing around this person in the middle of the night listening to his story. He has a doctor's appointment in the morning and would like a ride to the hospital. He feels fine and would just like a ride.

I explained to him, "You know, we have taxis."

"Oh no. Those cost money."

"Well, this ride costs twelve hundred just to step in the back."

He just stares at me, and I know he has no intention of paying any ambulance bill. Eventually, he called a cab.

We often have downtime and get bored. Up until now, the stories you have read have been completely true. I know this because I was there for each one. The few I will tell you next are stories that I heard from other firefighters. I believe them to be true because I know the people who told them and the people they involve.

Story One: The Dust Bunny

A good firefighter friend of mine, named Steve, has a bad case of sleep apnea. One quiet day at the fire station, he sits in the lounge chair and

John Wyatt

falls asleep, as he often does. He's famous for his ability to doze off in a matter of seconds. When I say he snores, I mean, he SNORES! Rafters shake, windows rattle, and women walking by the station grab their children and hurry past. Also working at the station is a crusty old engineer named Bud. The two are great friends and enjoy pulling pranks on each other. Bud being Bud, a diabolical prank hatches in his brain. Looking under the chairs, he finds a particularly large, hairy, dirty, nasty dust bunny. He picks it up with two fingers and moves the bunny back and forth over Steve's face, the wisps of nasty hair tickling the tip of his nose. Bursting awake, with hands flailing at his face, Steve sees Bud standing over him. "Get away!" he bellows and promptly falls back asleep. Bud is not so easily deterred. With an evil grin, he returns to dangling the bunny over his friend's face, only this time the entire mass suddenly disappears, like a rabbit down a hole. It's been sucked into Steve's nose and down his throat. He awakens a second time and begins to hack and gag like a big cat choking on a hairball.

True Stories from the Rolling Band-aid Box

"I said get away from me," he blurts out. The prankster is shocked and unsure of what to do. Steve settles back into the lazy boy chair and is soon back to counting sheep until his brain is startled awake by emergency tones blasting from the station loudspeakers for a cardiac arrest. Jumping up from his chair, he throws on his boots and rushes to the ambulance. Steve drives to the call and does his part to save a life. While transporting the patient to the hospital, he begins to cough and choke, feeling as though he is about to vomit up a lung. A rider who Steve is mentoring sits in the passenger seat of the cab, watching with concern. His convulsing body finally hacks up the dust bunny. Stopping the ambulance, he reaches into his mouth and finds the end of it. It has lost its dusty appearance and is now a long, wet, dirty, hairy mass. Holding the end, he slowly pulls a little over a foot of the nasty thing from his mouth until it hangs from his fingers in front of his face.

"What the hell?" he says.

This is just one of the stories that was told over and over at the dinner tables of our department. Firefighters love telling stories, and this one went far and wide.

Years later, the person who had been riding in the ambulance with Steve that day was now working on the other side of the country with FEMA in Florida. While chatting with a firefighter, she was asked if she had ever heard the story of the guy and the dust bunny. Amazed, she said, "Yes, he was one of my trainers." The Dust Bunny story has become one of Steve's claims to fame, and I am honored to share it with you.

Story Two: The Fire Hydrant

There is a monster of a man in the department who is so strong, it is said he could wrap his arms around a full refrigerator and move it aside by himself. We will call him Joe Firefighter. One dark night it is raining buckets, but this doesn't prevent Joe and his crew from being called to a house fire. Joe is the firefighter on the engine, and when they roll up to the house, his captain orders him to take the hydrant. This means that Joe was to jump out of the rig, walk to the back, grab the hydrant bag, remove the end of the five-inch hose from the hose bed, and attach it to the hydrant. That's exactly what he does, except for one small problem. As he approaches the hydrant, it moves, just a foot or so, but it moves. Joe stops in his tracks and stares.

It must be the rain, he thinks.

Dragging the hose behind him, he starts forward. The hydrant moves again. Joe stops and stares, not believing his eyes. Then, to his amazement, it turns and looks at him. His eyes go wide. It's a small boy in full yellow rain gear, including a rain hat that looks like the top of a fire hydrant.

Story Three: Out Fucking Standing

I reached out to the subject of this next story, and he gave permission for me to use his name, Shannon. He is a bear of a man who seems

John Wyatt

to walk the earth in total confidence, one of those guys who doesn't need to prove he's tough because everyone already knows he is. You might think a man like that would be scary, quite the opposite. Shannon has a ready grin that he shares easily with all his friends, of which there are many. When one of them would ask how he was doing, the answer was almost always, "Out fucking standing." At the age of five, Shannon's father gave him his first boxing gloves and taught his young son how to box. During his time in the military, Shannon put these skills to work fighting in matches called "Smokers." One day at the fire station, a friend of his slapped down a receipt on the table in front of him.

"I've signed you up for the Tough Guy tournament."

"What? he asked, feeling confused.

That's how he ended up in the ring facing the first of three opponents, a cocky ginger about twenty-two years old who was unaware of who he was facing. It didn't take long for him to find out. He spent most of the fight hiding in the corner, and Shannon won easily. The second fight was different. He faced a black belt in Karate, a very determined fighter who was not afraid to take a punch, and he took many of them. By the third round, Shannon had broken his nose and three ribs. The man was on his knees, holding one of Shannon's arms, refusing to give up. Shannon remembers hoping the referee would stop the fight because he didn't want to hurt the brave man anymore. The final was against a man about the same size as Shannon in weight and height, acting very confident and sporting a red Fu Manchu mustache. The bell rang, and both fighters came out swinging. Fu Manchu landed a couple of hard hits, and Shannon's head started to swim. Remembering back to his father's teaching, he covered up, protecting his head and ribs, and began to bob and weave. He let the now ineffective blows fall. Fu Manchu continued to swing wildly, and Shannon waited. In the third round, while against the ropes, the ref walked up to him and, placing a hand on his chest, asked Shannon, "Are you alright?

"Shit," was his reply.

Fu Manchu's attacks had become slower and weaker. His opponent had punched himself out, which is what Shannon had been waiting for. He began his assault and didn't stop until he won the fight. On that night, he became the Lane County Tough Guy champion and went out to eat pizza with friends and family. Like Shannon would say, "It was out fucking standing."

True Stories from the Rolling Band-aid Box

CHAPTER SIXTEEN

WOUNDED COWS

I would like to preface this story by saying I have nothing but respect for law enforcement. I came very close to becoming a police officer myself. Back before I became an EMT, after my discharge from the military, I had applied to the San Diego police department. Passing every hurdle, I had only to do the final Chief's interview. The possibility of becoming an officer of the law suddenly became very real. Did I really want to write tickets to speeders and work at a job where I had a target on my back, with the possibility of having to draw my weapon on someone? The more I thought about it, the more I decided it wasn't for me. As a firefighter, whenever I told people what I did for a living, they often said, "I could never do that, but I'm glad you can." I feel the same way about the police.

On this particular day, I'm the firefighter on an engine, part of a three-man crew. Receiving a call for a vehicle fire, we respond to a very rural area. Driving to the scene, we can see smoke rising in the distance. Pulling up, the engineer parks the engine on the grassy edge of the road near a small pickup fully engulfed in flames. Donning my gear, I pull the flaked hose out of a side bed onto the ground. The engineer charges the hose, and I begin putting water on the fire. Smoke and steam erupt from the vehicle as I move my hose stream over the hot metal. In no time, the flames are extinguished, and the vehicle is reduced to a smoking pile of stinking, burnt truck. I begin to pick up my equipment when a woman watching us work walks over to me.

"I know who started that fire," she says.

"Really, who's that?"

"The guy sitting under that tree," she says, pointing. "He says he's going to blow himself up."

"Really," I say, now very interested.

I report this information to my captain, a really nice guy and good friend, and he assesses the situation. Sitting perhaps sixty feet away, in a grassy field, is a man under a tree. He sits with his legs crossed, a five-gallon propane tank in his lap. The scene is very idyllic, with the sun shining on a small farmhouse, surrounded by a white picket fence, and cows munching on grass in the fields. The captain calls for a medic unit and police backup, then has the engineer move the engine up so it is directly across from the guy with the propane tank. I flak the hose next to the engine so that when he explodes into flames, I'll have a straight shot at him to put out the fire. It's best to be prepared. We wait and watch.

The police and medic unit arrive with noisy fanfare. Three plainclothes officers approach the man under the tree and speak with him for several minutes. Eventually, he rises and steps behind the tree. When he emerges, he's holding a rifle. Oh boy, plot twist. The officers draw their weapons, fan out around him, and begin yelling for him to drop the weapon. He casually walks out from under the branches of the tree, ignoring their orders. I'm frozen like a statue, watching the drama with wide eyes. Unknown to me, my captain has dropped to the ground and is crawling under the engine. In another life, he had been an Israeli commando and knew better than me the proper response to the situation. The man continues to walk, his rifle pointed at the ground, when the officers open fire. Standing fifteen feet from the police and forty feet from the guy with the rifle, I have a very good view of the incident. All three officers begin to rapid fire with their pistols, walking forward at the same time. Like a marionette whose strings are being pulled this way and that, he jerks each time he is hit. Once, twice, three times, a bullet strikes his body. He drops the rifle and falls to the ground, his strings cut. My medic instincts kick in, and I begin to walk toward the down man. An officer yells at me to stay back. They run to his side, move the rifle away and handcuff him. This done, they wave us over.

The medic crew is there with the gurney, and we all arrive at the patient's side together. One of the newer medics begins an assessment of the bleeding man. The other medic, a seasoned responder, and I lock eyes. Without talking, we both make the same decision in the blink of an eye. This guy needs a surgeon to survive, and anything else can be done in the back of the ambulance traveling Code 3 to the hospital. With no effort at being gentle, we grab him off the grass and place him on the gurney. I'm riding in the back of the medic unit, helping my fellow firefighter with patient care. When I have a moment, I ask our patient, "Hey buddy, what is going on with you?"

"Man, I'm having a bad day."

We found three bullet wounds in his body—three out of all the shots fired by the three officers. This made me wonder if maybe we should return later and look for wounded cows.

☙❧

Oregon is a wet state with lush forests, lakes, and rivers. We have the majority of our grass fires in the hot summer months when it's dryer. On one particularly hot day, a fire was started by a homeless camp. Winds were blowing hard, and the fire moved quickly across several acres of brown pasture. My crew responded in a brush rig—a specialized vehicle equipped with the tools to fight brush fires. We arrive at a spot downwind of the fire to prevent it from jumping the road. Grabbing a hose and nozzle, I move across a ditch filled with high dry grass and begin to prepare to fight the fire that is rapidly approaching. About this time, a newswoman arrives in her minivan. She jumps out in her knee-length skirt and four-inch heels, grabs a tripod with a camera mounted to it, and follows me into the field. Stepping like an excited deer in the high grass, she sets up her tripod right next to me. The fire is pushing towards us, and I'm still waiting for my engineer to send water to my nozzle.

I look at her and say, "I'm not sure that I'm going to be able to stop this fire." She looks at me with a puzzled expression then looks at the fire racing towards her. The alarm on her pretty face tells me the danger she's in has suddenly dawned on her. Quickly grabbing her tripod, she high steps back through the field, wobbles across the ditch and packs her equipment back into the minivan. The water arrives, and with the help of several more rigs and firefighters, we are able to stop the spread of the fire, saving an apartment complex in the process.

True Stories from the Rolling Band-aid Box

Just when you think you've seen everything, a call comes along to show you just how wrong you are. It's another bright and sunny morning. People are living their lives, riding bikes through the park, having a delightful breakfast with friends, maybe walking their dog along the river path. In one home, however, a woman calls 911 with a plea for help. Working the medic unit, we are dispatched to a nice house in a quiet neighborhood. I knock on the door. No answer, so I knock again and through the door hear the voice of a woman yelling from inside.

"I'm in here. Help!"

I try the door; it's locked.

"The door is locked," I yell.

"Help!"

This happens more often than you would think. We get "check patient calls" or respond to fire alarms when no one is home, and we have to break into a house. Hopefully, we find an unlocked window to crawl in, but sometimes we must break a window to make entry. On this call, a kitchen window is open, and my partner crawls through. He comes to the front door and lets me in. We find the poor woman in her bathroom. That same morning, she was released from the hospital after having abdominal surgery. She had gone to the bathroom to have a bowel movement, and her stitches had burst. So there she sits on the toilet, her lap covered in a steaming pile of pink, moist intestines. Totally conscious and unable to move, she looks at us in desperation. Not something you see every day.

I kneel next to her, place a hand on her shoulder and say, "Don't worry, I've got you."
My partner pulls a large trauma dressing out of the med box and wets it down with sterile saline. We wrap the intestines in this then secure the entire thing to her body with gauze. The transport was uneventful, and the woman was grateful, to say the least.

True Stories from the Rolling Band-aid Box

CHAPTER SEVENTEEN

THE IMPACT

As a firefighter and paramedic, I have been exposed to the horrors of what people do to themselves and others. Yet, the strength of the human mind can overcome even our strongest basic instincts, like self-preservation. This brings us to suicide. As you've read, I have witnessed hangings, shootings, even death by Drano. The most desperate, inventive, and stupid attempted suicide began one bright afternoon when everyone should have been giving thanks for being alive.

We respond to a 'man down' call in a remote area. It's a long response down a winding mountain road that ends at a tree-covered, dirt driveway. A two-story, rustic house comes into view with two Sheriff's vehicles parked in front. I exit the ambulance, and one of the officers comes to the second-story railing, looks down at me, and says, "You better get up here. It's bad."

I make my way into the home and up the steps to find a blood trail. Imagine you have a bucket of blood, splash a mop into it, then drag that mop through your house. I follow this wide red path down a hallway, stepping lightly, trying to avoid slipping in the wet mess. It leads to a room where two officers are standing above a man lying in a pool of gore. I can't help to notice the gaping, ragged wound that runs across his throat.

One of the Sheriffs looks at me and says, "He got his circular saw going and dropped it down across his neck. When it didn't kill him right away, he got scared, dragged himself in here, and called 911."

I kneel next to the patient to get a better look. He's conscious and calmly looking at me. The teeth of the spinning saw have done a lot of damage, opening his throat about ten inches, leaving shreds of flesh and muscle hanging in tatters. Yet, amazingly, I can see that his trachea, gleaming white in all that red mess, has not been damaged. He seems to be breathing easily. We quickly moisten a large trauma dressing and place it over the wound to slow the bleeding, then wrap gauze around his neck to keep it in place. We package him up for transport, and as we carry him out, I notice the saw that I had missed when we arrived. The power tool, covered in blood and pieces of flesh, is still plugged in. Out of all the ways to end your life, to lie on the floor and drop a spinning power saw on your neck seemed the craziest I have ever run across.

When death happens with family or friends in attendance, those people then become the patients. It's the survivors that need us after the sheet has been placed over the body. We console them and help with calling the appropriate authorities, often staying with them until someone else arrives. This is never more important than when the one that has passed is a child.

True Stories from the Rolling Band-aid Box

We are called to a home where CPR is being performed on an infant. The new parents had decided to place their newborn on the bed between them for the night. Unfortunately, one of them had unknowingly rolled onto it and smothered it in the process. Arriving, we find the infant lying on the carpet of the bedroom, a small trail of dried blood coming from its nose. The child is cold and gray, obviously having died an hour or more ago. The parents are standing over the body in shock, the mother crying uncontrollably.

I step up to the father. "I'm very sorry, but I believe your baby is gone."

"Please," he says, with tears in his eyes. "Can't you do anything?"

This is where things get difficult. The child is gone. Our patients are now this young mother and father who must live with what has happened the rest of their lives. As a crew, we decide to let them believe that everything possible was done to save their baby. Some people might argue that we gave them false hope. I would say that the false hope will only last a few minutes, while the knowledge that their child was given every chance will last a lifetime. We ran the code, doing CPR and giving a round of drugs. We then called a doctor, told him what had transpired, and he called the time of death. The husband thanked us for trying. The mother could only cry in his arms.

Some people have amazing willpower. I once found my younger brother in the garage, holding tightly to a vice that was bolted to the workbench. In his other hand was a sheet of heavy grit sandpaper. Years ago, he had gotten a tattoo on his forearm and had decided he no longer wanted it. There he was, crying, using the sandpaper to remove the unwanted ink. Blood is running down his arm, the pain unimaginable, but he would not stop—willpower.

True Stories from the Rolling Band-aid Box

Late at night, we are called to a home for bleeding. We are met at the door by a woman who tells us a strange woman showed up at her door asking for help. She lets us in and points to a woman sitting on a dining room chair in the middle of her living room. Her head is hanging down, dark black hair covers her face, and blood covers the front of her blouse. The woman sits silently as I walk up and kneel in front of her.

"Excuse me, ma'am, can you look up at me?" I ask quietly.

Slowly, she raises her head. Her eyes are wide but not as wide as the ragged gash that runs across her throat. Shreds of meat hang from the gaping wound, and blood oozes from torn flesh.

"How did this happen," I ask.

"He attacked me."

"Who did?"

"The man."

My partner calls for police backup while I assess and treat the patient. She's lucky that no major vessels were cut and survives the trip to the emergency room. Later, we are told that she has been admitted to the psych ward. They learned she had inflicted the wound to herself with a steak knife, slowly sawing it back and forth across her throat. She had done this hoping it would get her family's attention.

Most firefighters and EMS personnel will agree that the calls that result in a patient's life being saved are the most rewarding and tend to make up for all the soul-sucking, ridiculous, nonsense calls we respond to nearly every day. This was one of them for me. A driver is delivering a large order of bark mulch to a private home and parks his industrial size truck on a sloping driveway. After he exits the vehicle, it begins to slowly roll down the drive on its own. In alarm, he tries to climb back into the cab and grabs the steering wheel to pull himself in. Wrong move! The steering wheel turns, and the truck swings to the side, throwing the driver to the ground and tipping the truck onto its side. The homeowner hears the crash and runs outside to find the driver pinned under the massive bed of the vehicle. They call 911, and we respond with an ambulance, a truck, an engine, and a chief officer.

We find the driver, still pinned under the sidewall of the huge truck bed. Lying on his back in the dirt, his legs disappear under the heavy metal up to the middle of his thighs. The distance between the metal and the ground is only a few inches. His legs are crushed. Despite his injury, the patient is doing well. No other injuries are found or reported, and he is able to talk with us calmly. We know that this will not last because he will bleed to death the moment we lift the truck off him. We make a plan to save his life and go to work. I'm assigned patient care and start two large IVs so I can replace the fluid that will be lost. We place a C-collar on him and prepare the backboard and straps. The truck crew begins to dig on either side of the patient, where they will place the airbags. These are large square bags, incredibly tough, that can lift very heavy objects using compressed air. We also prepared the MAST pants. These trousers are like a large blood pressure cuff for your legs and abdomen. Our plan is to use them to control the bleeding that will occur when the weight is lifted off his legs.

Everything is ready, and we explain what is about to happen to the patient. He's scared but realizes it must be done. The air tanks are opened, the bags begin to fill, the truck begins to lift, and the patient begins to scream. The backboard is slid under him, and the legs of the MAST pants are placed on and inflated. Mercifully, he loses consciousness. With every bone in his legs shattered, his muscles contract, shortening his legs. Four of us ride in the back of the ambulance to work on him as we speed away. Our hard work and planning keep the patient alive, and that's the way we deliver him to the emergency room. We talk about the call in the medic room at the hospital while doing paperwork. We are all of the mind that he will lose both legs in surgery. Imagine our surprise when, a year later, he knocks on the door of our station house and walks in with a cane. We sat and talked for an hour. After several surgeries, the surgeons had been able to save both legs. We had been part of the team that saved his life and his legs. That is what the job is about—making a positive difference in people's lives. Even though many of my memories are dark and sad, they are offset by ones like this.

These are just a handful of the calls I have responded to in the thirty years I spent going to other people's emergencies. Many of them are not happy memories. People don't call 911 because they just got a new puppy; they call because they are in trouble and need help. I want to mention all the men and women who volunteer as firefighters and EMS personnel in their communities. They go to training, miss holidays with family, and drag themselves out of bed in the middle of the night to

John Wyatt

serve their neighbors without pay. They deserve our gratitude and respect. First responders feel a deep responsibility to deliver the best care and understand that this care affects thousands of lives. The job not only impacts our patients but their families, friends, and everyone they will meet in their lifetime. It was an honor to be part of the fire departments, ambulance crews, and teams that I worked with. I'm proud of my years as a first responder and will cherish them to my grave.

True Stories from the Rolling Band-aid Box